Tuberculosis and the
Politics of Exclusion

Critical Issues in Health and Medicine

Edited by Rima D. Apple, University of Wisconsin-Madison and Janet Golden, Rutgers University, Camden

Growing criticism of the U.S. health care system is coming from consumers, politicians, the media, activists, and health care professionals. Critical Issues in Health and Medicine is a collection of books that explores these contemporary dilemmas from a variety of perspectives, among them political, legal, historical, sociological, and comparative, and with attention to crucial dimensions such as race, gender, ethnicity, sexuality, and culture.

Tuberculosis and the Politics of Exclusion

A History of Public Health and Migration to Los Angeles

Emily K. Abel

Rutgers University Press

New Brunswick, New Jersey, and London

Library of Congress Cataloging-in-Publication Data

Abel, Emily K.
  Tuberculosis and the politics of exclusion : a history of public health and
  migration to Los Angeles / Emily K. Abel.
      p. ;   cm. — (Critical issues in health and medicine)
  Includes bibliographical references and index.
  ISBN 978-0-8135-4175-4 (hardcover : alk. paper) —
  ISBN 978-0-8135-4176-1 (pbk. : alk. paper)
    1. Tuberculosis—California—Los Angeles—History—19th century.
    2. Tuberculosis—Califonia—Los Angeles—History—20th century.
    3. Immigrants—Diseases—California—Los Angeles—History—19th century.
    4. Immigrants—Diseases—California—Los Angeles—History—20th century.
    5. Immigrants—Medical care—California—Los Angeles—History—19th century.
    6. Immigrants—Medical care—California—Los Angeles—History—20th century.
    7. Discrimination in medical care—California—Los Angeles—History—19th century.
    8. Discrimination in medical care—California—Los Angeles—History—20th century.
    9. Public health—California—Los Angeles—History—19th century.
  10. Public health—California—Los Angeles—History—20th century.
  11. Los Angeles (Calif.)—Ethnic relations—History—19th century.
  12. Los Angeles (Calif.)—Ethnic relations—History—20th century.
  I. Title. II. Series.
  [DNLM: 1. Tuberculosis, Pulmonary—history—Los Angeles.   2. History, 19th Century—
  Los Angeles.   3. History, 20th Century—Los Angeles.   4. Minority Groups—Los Angeles.
  5. Prejudice—Los Angeles.   6. Public Health—history—Los Angeles. WF 300 A139t 2007]
  RC313.C2A25   2007
  616.9'9500979494—dc22   2007000028

A British Cataloging-in-Publication record for this book is available from the British Library.

Visit our Web site: http://rutgerspress.rutgers.edu

Manufactured in the United States of America

Contents

Illustrations

Acknowledgments

Many people read all or part of the manuscript, including Rick Abel, Karen Brodkin, Janet Brodie, Amy Fairchild, Sharla Fett, Janet Golden, Rachel Lee, Natalia Molina, Doreen Valentine, Devra Weber, and Alice Wexler. Douglas Flamming directed me to relevant documents. Sabah Uddin and Ellie Hickerson provided research assistance. Archivists who rendered essential help included Robert G. Marshall of the Urban Archives Center, California State University, Northridge; Katharine E. S. Donahue, Teresa G. Johnson, and Russell A. Johnson, all of the History Division, UCLA Louise M. Darling Biomedical Library; Dace Taube, Regional History Curator, Specialized Libraries and Archival Collections, University of Southern California; and Bill Frank, Curator of Hispanic, Cartographic, and Western Historical Manuscripts at the Huntington Library.

I received permissions from the Huntington Library, San Marino, California, to quote from the Charles Willard Collection and the John Anson Ford Collection; from the Specialized Libraries and Archival Collections, Doheny Memorial Library, University of Southern California, Los Angeles, to quote from the Records of the Chamber of Commerce and from the oral history interview with Zdenka Buben; from the Center for Oral and Public History, California State University, Fullerton, to quote from oral history interviews; from the Department of Special Collections, Young Research Library, University of California, Los Angeles, to quote from the George Pigeon Clements Collection and the Los Angeles Urban League Papers; from Sheila Rhoads, to quote from the interview with David Lubin; from the Kansas State Historical Society, Topeka, Kansas, to quote from the Martha Shaw Farnsworth Collection; from the Urban Archives Center, Oviatt Library, Northridge, California, to quote from the Jewish Family Service Society of Los Angeles Collection and the Greater Los Angeles Visitors and Convention Bureau Collection; from the Breathe California of Los Angeles County to quote from the Report of the Directors, Los Angeles Tuberculosis and Health Association; and from Cathryn Griffith, to quote from the diary of Margaret Love Stone.

The book was supported by the UCLA Chicano Studies Research Center and by grant number 5G13LM007969 from the National Library of Medicine. The contents are solely my responsibility and do not necessarily represent the official views of the Chicano Studies Research Center or the National Library of Medicine. Portions of chapters 3 and 6 appeared in "From Exclusion to

Expulsion: Mexicans and Tuberculosis Control in Los Angeles, 1914–1940," *Bulletin of the History of Medicine*, v. 77, no. 4 (Winter 2003): 823–49 and " 'Only the Best Class of Immigration': Public Health Policy toward Mexicans and Filipinos in Los Angeles, 1910–1940," *American Journal of Public Health*, v. 94, no. 6 (June 2004): 932–939.

As always, my family provided the love and support on which I depend.

Tuberculosis and the Politics of Exclusion

Introduction

Arriving in Los Angeles in the early 1930s, "noir" writer Louis Adamic found sickness everywhere. Unlike his native Slovenia, where "good health was the rule, rather than the exception . . . and so there was little interest in it," the Southern California city had so many invalids that health was "the leading topic of conversation."[1] Adamic's primary goal was to debunk the myths circulated by city boosters. Although notorious for its polluted air today, Los Angeles once billed itself as a health resort, especially for people with "lung troubles." Soon after the arrival of the transcontinental railroad in 1876, publicists had launched a massive crusade to portray the metropolis as the promised land and circulated countless stories of miraculous cures. A poem in one of the first issues of a prominent booster journal claimed that "pleasure, toil, and rest, alike bestow/On mind and body—the vigor, strength, and health."[2] The author of a prize-winning letter published in the journal had come to Los Angeles "a physical wreck—pale, haggard, and debilitated," but had quickly "been restored" and was now "simply robust."[3]

Adamic was hardly the first to emphasize the enormous gap between the city's glittering image and its darker reality. Because the inflated booster rhetoric promised more than could possibly be delivered, the city soon contained an unusually large proportion of sick and dying people. Tuberculosis (or consumption, as it was often called) was especially prevalent. The most fearsome disease of the time, TB is an ancient scourge which we now know is caused by the tubercle bacillus. A latent form of disease develops as soon as the microbe enters the body; active illness is most likely to occur in bodies weakened by inadequate diets, other health problems, stress, and poor living conditions. At the turn of the twentieth century, some people enjoyed remissions of years and occasionally even decades after the appearance of symptoms, but permanent cure was impossible until the 1946 advent of antibiotics. Many declarations of recovery in the California sunshine thus proved premature. Long before Adamic's arrival, visitors complained about the ubiquity of tuberculosis. As early as the 1890s one victim of the disease in Los Angeles wrote that he encountered a fellow sufferer "at every street corner."[4] A woman who accompanied her consumptive brother-in-law reported that they "constantly" met other invalids.[5]

What is most striking about Adamic's account is not his focus on the illness the boosters camouflaged but rather the extent to which he shared their basic assumptions. By exalting good health and making recovery the only permissible outcome, city publicists had denigrated people who did not get well. Those with advanced disease and the most conspicuous symptoms attracted particularly fierce condemnation. A similar hostility toward invalids pervaded Adamic's writings. As he acknowledged, "ill-looking people generally affect me unpleasantly." Explaining his move from downtown to San Pedro, he wrote, "It looked sane. There were no tourists and sick old people. . . . It was a normal seaport town."[6] Like the boosters he pilloried, Adamic believed that sickness and old age were disgusting and abnormal and could be eradicated.

Those attitudes shaped L.A.'s response to the widespread tuberculosis in its midst. After wooing health seekers from the East, the metropolis adopted a politics of exclusion, erecting numerous barriers to entry. As in East Coast cities at the turn of the twentieth century, health officials emphasized the prevalence of the disease among immigrants, depicted them as agents rather than victims of disease, and called for border control. But the tuberculosis story unfolded differently in Los Angeles for several reasons. One was that members of the white elite were especially ready to embrace an exclusionary strategy because they viewed themselves as a uniquely blessed people; they could sustain an illusion of invulnerability only by banishing anyone identified with weakness and danger.

In addition, partly as a result of the widespread publicity campaign, migrants poured into Los Angeles not only from other countries but also from the eastern United States. The first exclusionary drive mounted by public health officials focused on white, single men labeled "tramps" during the 1890s and early 1900s. When a bill to establish a statewide quarantine failed, officials sought to prevent the influx of consumptives in other ways. State authorities sponsored a federal bill to discourage low-income people with tuberculosis from leaving the East and dispatched posters to train stations throughout the country, warning that California provided no free care to residents of other states. Charitable groups urged East Coast branches to stop sending people with tuberculosis to the West and refused to assist those who arrived. Anxieties about attracting the "wrong kind" of people also retarded government efforts to care for tuberculosis sufferers. The first attempt to establish a public sanatorium met defeat largely because of fears that it would attract impoverished health seekers. Proposals to enlarge the county hospital, housing the sickest TB patients, provoked a similar outcry. And a campaign to create a Jewish sanatorium elicited the complaint that the city could become "the mecca for indigent tubercular patients."[7] Although both government authorities and local advocates eventually established a broad range of free and low-cost tuberculosis services, Los Angeles lagged far behind East Coast municipalities.[8]

Another distinctive feature of Los Angeles is that the major immigrant group came from Mexico rather than eastern and southern Europe. Some Mexicans entered Southern California during the 1900s and 1910s, but most arrived during the 1920s, by which time immigration from Europe had greatly diminished. Because many worked in agriculture rather than in industry, they were assumed to pose a grave threat to the food supply. They also encountered uncompromising discrimination. While European immigrants gradually came to be seen as white, Mexicans increasingly were racialized as brown. Segregation was common in education, health care, and public accommodations throughout Los Angeles County. And nativists sought not just to restrict the entry of Mexicans during the 1920s but also to expel them during the 1930s. State and local health officials were major players in the deportation and repatriation drives, which reduced the size of the Mexican community in Los Angeles by a third. The association of tuberculosis thus had an even more devastating impact on Mexicans in that city than on the European immigrants in the East Coast whom many medical historians previously have examined. Growing fears about the resurgence of the disease, especially among "new" immigrant groups, endow this topic with enormous significance. As in the early twentieth century, anti-immigration groups repeatedly charge that immigrants import dread diseases into the country and impose unbearable burdens on the health care system.

After the expulsion of Mexicans, health officials turned their attention to Filipinos, again urging those with tuberculosis to depart and providing transportation home. A far more extensive campaign targeted the thousands of people who poured into Los Angeles from other parts of the nation. Inspiring both Woody Guthrie's protest songs and John Steinbeck's 1939 *Grapes of Wrath*, those "inter-state migrants" reported serious physical problems, including tuberculosis. Health authorities thus participated enthusiastically in efforts to seal the city's borders, even lending support to Police Chief Davis's notorious "bum brigade." As the financial crisis deepened, exclusion shaded easily into expulsion. Migrants with TB who applied for financial assistance or medical care received only train fare out of the metropolis.

Finally, the especially virulent animus toward long-term invalids in Los Angeles highlights the chronic nature of tuberculosis. The disease not only killed more people than any other malady but also disabled its victims for months and often years. A host of recent studies has enormously enlarged our understanding of how the discovery of the tubercle bacillus and the gradual acceptance of the germ theory transformed the medical treatment, social situation, and cultural representation of sufferers between 1880 and 1940.[9] A Los Angeles perspective reminds us that the stigma surrounding tuberculosis stemmed not only from the new bacteriological knowledge but also from a distaste for physical difference. People with advanced disease were especially likely to be shunned because they displayed symptoms that violated reigning standards of how bodies should look and act. Moreover, the primary justification for expelling tubercular Mexicans during the 1930s was not that they spread the disease to the white population but rather that, because they remained sick for so long, they overwhelmed public resources by consuming extensive amounts of monetary assistance and medical services. That argument had special cogency when the Great Depression forced state and local authorities to slash programs and growers agitated for open borders by contending that Mexicans represented a cheap labor force.

Low-income sufferers of tuberculosis responded to the public health program in various ways. Once services became available, some patients lined up to receive clinic care, assiduously followed medical recommendations, and gratefully accepted placement in hospitals and sanatoriums. Many others, however, disregarded clinic appointments, rejected advice, and either failed to enroll in institutions or fled soon after arrival. The exclusionary campaign elicited equally divergent reactions. Although some Mexicans, Filipinos, and "interstate migrants" welcomed the opportunity to leave Los Angeles during the 1930s, most resisted expulsion. And a few groups and individuals powerfully challenged prevailing assumptions about who should be considered a burden and who a resource, asserting their right not only to remain in the metropolis but also to share equally in its social and economic benefits.

Chapter 1

Pestilence in the Promised Land

Nineteenth-century Americans considered themselves a uniquely blessed people, exempt from the normal vicissitudes of life. Alexis de Tocqueville famously found the country "a course almost without limits, a field without horizon," a place where "the human spirit rushes forward . . . in every direction."[1] And the West was the epitome of American promise, the destination of all easterners in search of regeneration and renewal. Consumptives figured prominently among those travelers. Since ancient times, it had been widely believed that certain air, soil, and water could promote health. Westward journeys in search of cures for lung problems began in the early 1800s, stopped temporarily during the Civil War, and then rapidly increased in number after fighting ended.[2] Health seekers sent back glowing accounts of eating and sleeping outdoors, riding horses, and hunting buffalo, conquering disease while conquering other forms of nature.[3]

After the extension of the Southern Pacific Railroad from San Francisco to Los Angeles in 1876, Southern California towns and cities began to vie for the invalid trade by touting the remarkable curative power of the climate and the newly planted citrus orchards. Trying to counter the image of hardship, adventure, and danger traditionally associated with the West, boosters assured consumptives they could live in comfort and ease. In his 1885 *Homes and Happiness in the Golden State of California*, Benjamin Cummings Truman wrote that "no State in the Union spends more relatively on its common schools, or has a better educational system or more competent teachers."[4] Other literature claimed that the many elegant hotels that dotted the landscape obviated the need for "roughing it."[5] Even new settlers could find large, beautiful homes, rather than the crude shacks of many frontier areas. Work in the orange groves was "healthful" and "light."[6]

But if invalids were now encouraged to achieve cure by living harmoniously with nature rather than by wrestling with it, the basic message remained the same—recovery was available to anyone who sought it. I. M. Holt, the secretary of the Immigration Association of San Bernardino County, declared Southern California "Nature's Great Sanitarium."[7] A former invalid proclaimed, "Steady, persistent cultivation of the soil, in a pure atmosphere and under a genial sky, like we have here, will as surely save from destruction any lungs capable of salvation, as faith will save the soul."[8] An article in a prominent booster journal asserted, "A consumptive who can live in sunshine year in and year out has chances for life not obtainable under other conditions." The author believed that "California sunshine has helped keep him alive and arrest the ravages of disease which threatened him with death within a few years."[9] Statistics gave the patina of science to such claims. According to an editorial entitled "Living on Climate," "There are some thirty or forty thousand people in Southern California who were doomed to death in the eastern climate, and are allowed under these balmy skies to continue their lives to old age."[10]

Recovery was promised metaphorically as well as literally. Writer after writer gave examples of plants or flowers that barely survived in the East but flourished in Southern California. Although "the apricot in every other locality except California is of delicate growth and requires much care and nursing to bring it to maturity, here it ranks in hardiness with the peach and requires no more attention than it."[11] The calla lily was "a dwarfish plant which the housewife in the East nurses in its little pot in a warm room to coax its feeble blossom," but "it grows here out of doors the year round."[12]

The other side of celebrating good health was blaming those who did not get well. Once recovery became the only permissible outcome, sufferers increasingly met hostility. Successful health seekers often presented their new robustness as a sign of superiority and described long-term invalids as hopeless and resigned. George F. Weeks provides a case in point. A New York journalist, Weeks was twenty four in 1876 when his weight plummeted and paroxysms of coughing began to overwhelm him. He consulted Dr. Austin Flint, a well-known physician, who diagnosed consumption and recommended that Weeks leave the dangerous urban air. His destination was a a sanatorium in San Bernardino, California, but it quickly repelled him. Rather than actively pursuing a cure, he and the other residents "sat about the fire, gloomy, despondent, and disheartened, stewing in the poisons of our own emanations, waiting for what most of us knew was coming."[13] He thus fled after one night, finding work on a cattle and bee ranch. Stoically denying his physical pain, he slept outside, rode wild horses, shot bears and mountain lions, stole irrigation water, and tricked

Indians. Within a few months he was well enough to resume his newspaper career and send for his family.

In preparation for their arrival, he laid claim to a shack on a plot of land abandoned "by another One-Lunger who had waited too long before coming to this Land of New Lungs, and whose weary bones were resting on the hillside beyond the Sanitarium."[14] Having won the race for survival, Weeks was entitled to all the rewards. Three years later he looked "well tanned, full of life and vigor" and weighed "a normal 165 or 170 pounds" for his "six feet of stature."[15] In the portrait he chose for the frontispiece of his 1928 autobiography, he stands with his arms crossed, legs apart, and posture erect—the iconic pose of Theodore Roosevelt, the embodiment of the victorious western hero.

A health seeker who recorded his experiences in far greater detail, Charles D. Willard had a more complicated relationship to the narrative of recovery. Like Weeks, Willard worked for many years as a journalist, was diagnosed with tuberculosis in his early twenties, received advice to leave unhealthy urban air, and settled first in San Bernardino. But there the resemblance ended. The dominant themes of the letters he sent to his family in Chicago are painful dislocation, anxiety, and loss, not regeneration and triumph over all adversity. When he arrived in Southern California in 1886, he was so sick he had to be carried off the train. Although he occasionally enjoyed long periods of remission, married, raised a child, engaged in various forms of employment, and rose to prominence in Los Angeles civic and political life, the specter of a relapse relentlessly haunted him. In 1914, he died of the disease that had sent him from home nearly three decades earlier.[16]

Erving Goffman writes that the standards the "stigmatized individual" has "incorporated from the wider society equip him to be intimately alive to what others see as his failing."[17] Willard not only absorbed prevailing attitudes; he also helped to write the cultural script. As secretary of the Los Angeles Chamber of Commerce between 1891 and 1897, he spearheaded the activities that helped to make Los Angeles one of the best advertised American cities. His central message was that the metropolis was the promised land, where everyone could find robust good health. Acutely aware of the exalted value attached to strength and vigor, Willard carefully concealed his illness in public. He allowed none of his chamber colleagues to perceive the infirmities that constricted his life. Donning elegant clothes to hide his emaciation, he described himself for many years as a sufferer of neurasthenia, a widespread but less dreaded affliction. When he no longer could disguise his diagnosis, he tried to conceal the likelihood that it soon would prove fatal. Appointed editorial consultant to the major journal of the California progressive movement five years before his death, he crafted the persona of a forceful and determined political writer.[18]

Willard was hardly alone in writing triumphalist narratives while hiding all evidence of sickness. Frank Wiggins worked closely with Willard at the Chamber of Commerce and assumed his position as secretary in 1897.[19] Wiggins, too, had arrived in Southern California in 1886 so ill with consumption he left the train on a stretcher.[20] In a published history of the Chamber of Commerce, Willard described his former partner thus: "For sometime it was an open question whether recovery was possible, but at last the climate performed the same miracle that it has accomplished in thousands of other cases, and Mr. Wiggins was ready to throw his tremendous energies into new work under new skies."[21] Another historian wrote, "There probably is no more striking individual example of the possibilities of Southern California from the standpoint of health and human development than Mr. Wiggins."[22] Nevertheless, Wiggins failed to display the signs of robust well-being that he urged the public to associate with Los Angeles. Newspaper cartoons during the 1890s ridiculed his thin frame and stooped shoulders.[23] In a somewhat bizarre attempt at humor, the toastmaster at the 1899 chamber annual dinner stated, "When God made man, he made him large—large as a mountain in comparison to a grain of sand; but when he made the Siamese twins of the Chamber of Commerce, Willard and Wiggins, he ran out of material and endowed them as thin as living skeletons."[24]

Although not a consumptive, Charles Fletcher Lummis had considerable difficulty fulfilling the image of vigor and vitality he helped to create. After a stint as city editor of the Los Angles Times, he assumed control of The Land of Sunshine, a booster journal Willard had founded. Introducing Lummis to his readers in 1894, Willard wrote, "Unlike many men who are known to the world through their brains, Mr. Lummis has a powerful physique and rejoices in its exercise."[25] His mode of transportation had announced his unusual strength. Disdaining the trains carrying invalids to the city, Lummis departed from Ohio on foot. And his famous account of his walk emphasized the many ways he differed from the "poor health seeker." He was "perfectly well and a trained athlete," able to overcome all physical annoyances.[26] After "trudging across the corner of Ohio" and the "whole length of Indiana and Illinois," enormous blisters covered his feet. "But the experienced walker does not nurse such blisters," he insisted

If you sit down and cure them, they come back as soon as you resume the march. If you will shut your teeth and trudge on, and bear the extreme pain for a few days, the rebellious soles gradually toughen into self-cure, and the cure is permanent throughout the journey. So I limped ahead, with very sorry grimaces and a sorrier gait, but without giving up, and by the time I stood in Missouri my feet were as happy as all the rest of my body. A strain of my ankle just as starting cured itself in the same way.[27]

The longer he tramped, the stronger he became; by Colorado he had "grown robust as a young bison."[28] Four years after arriving in Los Angeles, however, Lummis had a major stroke; two smaller ones occurred during his long recovery in New Mexico.[29] Although he eventually was able to return to Los Angeles and become a cultural leader, he may well have remained aware that good health is always provisional.

A common assumption is that Los Angeles boosters were primarily men who arrived as invalids, rapidly regained their health, and sought to share their good fortunes with others.[30] But Willard, Wiggins, and Lummis tell a different story. Far from drawing on their success in surmounting all difficulties, they appear to have expressed their own yearnings for rejuvenation. The weakness and fragility they most urgently needed to camouflage were their own.

The railroads brought not only middle-class health seekers the boosters wooed but also many poorer ones, who became synonymous with "tramps" and thus met a much cooler reception. The "tramp scare" that spread through the United States bore many elements of a "moral panic"—exaggerated media reports, the conflation of a targeted group with danger, and calls for aggressive forms of social control.[31] The anxiety focused on tramps had a certain irony in a city attempting to create itself by attracting migrants. The biographer of a prominent tuberculosis physician explained why he sought recovery from the disease between 1909 and 1914 first in Colorado Springs, Colorado, then in Cheyenne, Wyoming, then in Kingston, Tucson, and then in Castle Hot Springs, Arizona, before finally reaching Los Angeles. "In those days it was literally 'chasing the cure,' for it was thought that if you could find the right climate for your particular case you would soon get well."[32] But as one historian reminds us, although mobility is a vaunted American ideal, some people "are supposed to know their place."[33] Indigent consumptives rarely were described as traveling purposefully; instead, they "roamed," "drifted," and "wandered." In 1915 a former surgeon in the U.S. Public Health Service explained that because poor people, were "dissatisfied and poorly contented . . . many of them even after their arrival in a favorable climate wander from place to place in search of better conditions."[34] And some indigent consumptives were diagnosed with "wanderlust," a new pathological condition requiring the victim to move incessantly.[35] In 1917, the physician at a Los Angeles chest clinic reported that many of his patients "left for Arizona within three weeks of the time that I saw them, on their own initiative, not by my advice, and I have found that most of these cases are troubled, particularly if they are men, with the wanderlust, and do not stay sufficiently long to get a concise record or adequate treatment."[36]

Prominent boosters helped to sound the alarm about both tramps in general and the consumptives among them. In 1895 the Chamber of Commerce declared, "Our city is infested with hobos, tramps, beggars and other impecunious persons who are rendering themselves obnoxious and have become a dangerous element to the peace of the city." The City Council should establish barracks where "such persons" would be required to work in return for lodging and food.[37] As chamber secretary, Charles D. Willard transcribed such sentiments; when he left that post, he sought to spread them more broadly. Soon after his appointment as the editor of a major local newspaper in 1897, he wrote, "It is to the interest of the entire community that the tramp nuisance should be abolished." Because "Southern California has a winter climate which will always attract visitors of an undesirable class," Los Angeles would always have a "tramp problem." He demanded that the police stop its practice of providing free lodging.[38] "Placing these fellows in jail during the winter months suits them too well. The jail is fairly comfortable and the meals come regularly." The "only feasible plan" was to force vagrants to work at "the rock pile" to earn their keep.[39]

Willard continued the antitramp campaign when he became secretary of the Municipal League, the city's major progressive organization, in 1901. One of his first tasks was to travel to various midwestern cities to investigate their reform movements. On his return, he wrote approvingly of laws in Wisconsin and Minnesota "fining railroads for bringing indigent invalids over the border"[40] and urged Los Angeles to institute "rigid inspection of private lodging houses by the police" under the guise of sanitary regulations. Willard concluded that tramps represented "the great national disease"; charity dispensed outside punitive institutions served to nourish "this pestilence."[41] Tramps thus not only carried consumption, they also personified it. They constantly menaced, could erupt at any time, and needed firm control.

Who were the men who inspired such fear and loathing? Many probably were unskilled, seasonal workers. One historian estimates that "between 10 and 20 percent of the U.S. population in the late nineteenth century came from families with a member who had tramped in search of work."[42] Migrant laborers were overwhelmingly native born, single men, between the ages of twenty and forty.[43] Traveling by rail, they congregated in cities at the end of the line. Many field hands who produced the oranges advertised so effectively by the chamber followed the crops from orchard to orchard during the growing season before repairing to Los Angeles for the winter months.[44]

The bodies they were most likely to harm were their own. Riding the rails was, in a historian's words, "perilous business." Workers

> suffocated in the engine gases of slow freights in long tunnels, died in train wrecks, and were swept off or decapitated by low trestles, walkways, and bridges. Sleeping in the sun while riding the tops of swaying boxcars, they rolled down the pitched roofs and off into space. . . . Seated in a box-car doorway, they had their legs amputated when the train lurched and the big doors snapped shut like a guillotine. Curled up in a pile of straw at one end of a boxcar full of lumber, they were smeared against the bulk-head when rough switching in the yards or heavy application of the air brakes catapulted the lumber load against and through the car ends. . . . Others died after being trapped inside empty refrigerator cars.[45]

Still others died from jumping off trains or beatings by railway authorities. Exhaustion, poor food, and wretched accommodations left workers vulnerable to a range of diseases, including tuberculosis. Most were old by the age of forty.[46]

While some commentators identified indigent consumptives with tramps and danger, others employed a very different rhetoric. Perhaps a desire to portray themselves as benevolent rescuers motivated several doctors and reformers to describe poor people with TB as a pitiful group. "Unfortunate, deluded crea-tures,"[47] they typically waited so long to come to Southern California that they arrived long after they might have been able to benefit from the climate. Although all had "exhausted their slender means coming to this State,"[48] none was strong enough to work. They thus were compelled to sleep in poorly ventilated lodging houses and eat in cheap restaurants, receiving neither the sunshine nor the nourishing food believed necessary for recovery.[49] "Far from home, friends, and comforts,"[50] they suffered from "homesickness" and longed "for the tender ministrations of friends."[51] A few were lucky enough to find refuge in the county hospital. Many others died alone, "strangers in a strange world."[52]

The image of the single man dying by himself in a cheap lodging house was repeated so often that it became the conventional wisdom. Some evidence sug-gests, however, that this portrait too was deceptively simple. One historian con-cludes that tramp life "bred close, if temporary, friendships. On the road, men frequently formed partnerships for reasons of safety, frugality, and company. . . . In a world of strangers, migrants drew upon their class experiences to impro-vise new forms of obligation and mutual aid."[53] We can assume that at least some sick lodging-house residents were able to draw on that "ethic of reciproc-ity and mutualism."[54]

The diary of Martha Shaw further complicates the picture. A Kansas woman, Martha had been married to Johnny Shaw, a postman, for two months in November 1897, when he began to display disturbing symptoms, and doctors suspected consumption. During the next five years he tried various remedies, including a seven-week stay in a Chicago hospital and two extended trips to Colorado. Finally, on December 19, 1892, the couple boarded the Santa Fe Railroad, arriving in Los Angeles two days later.[55]

According to Martha, they "awakened" the next morning to "green lawns, bright flowers, trees in fruit and bloom: the fragrance of Orange blossoms, and the songs of birds, in the air: a blue sky and bright sunshine over all." Johnny was "delighted with all this Tropical beauty."[56] Best of all, his symptoms abated. Martha was able to report on January 10, 1893, that he "gains about a pound a week," on the 15th that "he grows stronger," and on the 17th that "he continues to improve in health."[57] Because he remained too sick to work, Martha found a job as a waitress in a hotel, but he was well enough to join her on various excursions. Sunday, January 8, was "such a beautiful day" that they "went for a walk up to the Water-works Reservoir on the high hills North of us."[58] On February 18, they "went down thro' Chinatown," where they were "very courteously treated, everywhere, to tea, candies, fruits and nuts."[59] After lunch the following week, the couple "took a car out to West Lake Park: a *very* pretty place."[60]

When Martha was at work, Johnny explored on his own. "Johnny goes out and is getting some acquainted," Martha wrote in January.[61] The following month she noted, "Johnny likes to go to the different Lunch-rooms and buy his meals and does so, many times and seems to enjoy it very much. Almost every block has a Hotel, Boarding House, Lunch room or pretty, little Delicacy Store, where one can get dainty, tempting meals as cheaply as to get at home."[62]

Only the weather displeased. "So much rainy weather very hard on Johnny," Martha wrote in February.[63] As his health began to deteriorate in early spring, they both blamed the persistent chill. On March 21, Martha "came home after Lunch, for Johnny is not at all well."[64] Soon afterwards, he rejected an invitation to go to the beach, "fearing it will be too cold for him."[65] But despite poor health, his social life expanded. On March 27, Martha noted that he went "everyday to the Fire Station across the street to sit in the sun and visit the Firemen."[66] On April 9, she described new neighbors "in our Flat, Mr. George Hill and sister and a Mr. William Thayer and young son, Louville."[67] Four days later Mr. Thayer "put a Telegraph Instrument in our room and strung wires to the Instrument in his rooms and is teaching Johnny 'Telegraphy' just to 'pass time' and to occupy him, when too stormy to be out doors."[68] Early in May, "Mr. Thayer and Louville spent [the] evening with us, Mr. Thayer bringing his violin and giving us some nice music."[69] On June 11, Martha remained at work all day "since Johnny can visit neighbor Thayer who plays violin for him."[70]

Although Johnny accompanied Martha to a "Ball game at Athletic Park" on June 16, the weather continued to take its toll.[71] "*Very, awful, fog* today," Martha wrote the following day, "and the consequent, heavy air, *very hard* on Johnny."[72] On June 26, he was "so weak" he could "get no farther than across the street on his walks."[73] On July 3 he was "anxious to go home, thinking if he gets away from this damp climate he will get well."[74] He declined to participate in the Fourth of July celebration the following day because he was "too weak to be out in the night air."[75]

By the end of July, Martha had "quit work" and was "home to stay, for Johnny has grown so much worse, it is not safe to leave him alone any more."[76] She had various forms of support. On July 15 she returned "some dishes" to a friend who had "brought some dainty food to Johnny—everyone is so kind to us."[77] An entry two days later read: "My friends send many things to Johnny." One gave Martha "a bottle of fine wine to take home to him." Others brought "fruits and flowers."[78] Johnny's friends rendered another type of care. "Henry Augustine, one of the Firemen, in station across the street, came in to see Johnny this afternoon," Martha wrote on July 27.[79]

There were several news items for August 1. A letter from Johnny's mother brought "money to go home on"; "Mrs. Barkey and Mrs. Sweezey, both former Topekans, to whom Johnny used to carry mail, called this morning to see us, having just found out we were here"; and Martha "called at Mrs. Cook's (also a former Topekan)" before making "final arrangements for our trip home."[80] The following day various people, including Henry Augustine, arrived to say good-bye. "Mrs. Sweezey and Mrs. Barkey came with a large lunch basket, filled with a nice Lunch and fine fruit" and went to the station "to see us off." Mrs. Cook "came with her carriage, to take us to the Depot." There the conductor picked Johnny "up in his arms and carried him into the train."[81] He died in Topeka three months later.[82]

Like the tubercular poor who dominated the writings of late-nineteenth-century commentators, Johnny was so sick when he reached Los Angeles that he could no longer work. But he challenged the dominant portrait of low-income people with tuberculosis in two critical ways: first, because he came with his wife, he could rely on her earnings. If he never achieved the affluence of the migrants wooed by boosters, he was hardly as poor as the indigent consumptive they despised. The notion of a rigid dichotomy between desirable and undesirable health seekers underlay both the exclusionary policies public health authorities enthusiastically embraced and the services they reluctantly established. Johnny Shaw's experience reminds us that at least some consumptives could not fit into either group.

Second, Johnny rarely was alone, even when his wife was away. A sociable man, he started to get "acquainted" soon after arriving. When too sick to venture out, he received visits from a fireman stationed across the street and neighbors in his own block of flats. Common ties of home also assuaged his loneliness. Two Topeka acquaintances provided a carriage for the trip to the station and food for the long return journey. His major complaint was the enormous discrepancy between the constant sunshine the boosters promised and the dismal rain and chill of a Los Angeles winter.

Health seeking was clearly an overwhelmingly male enterprise.[83] The three individuals who described their recoveries in inflated terms (Willard, Wiggins, and Lummis) were men. Men also dominated the ranks of low-income health seekers, whether depicted as dangerous tramps or pitiful invalids. Other evidence comes from the testimony of a woman who accompanied her consumptive brother-in-law to Los Angeles in 1876. "Since coming here," Jennie Collier wrote, "We have met more invalid men than women. It is more probable that men are more disposed to seek a change of climate for health than women."[84]

The records of the few institutions serving indigent people with tuberculosis also reveal a predominance of men. According to a survey of the tuberculosis records of Los Angeles County Hospital, men represented 699 (nearly 80 percent) of the 845 consumptives discharged during the first eleven months of 1912.[85] Although they come somewhat later, the records of a major philanthropy provide further insight. I examined all cases of tubercular migrants who applied for assistance from the Jewish Social Service Bureau (later the Jewish Family Service Society of Los Angeles) between 1926 and 1937. Those records indicate marital status as well as gender. Roughly similar numbers of men and women had arrived with spouses (six men and five women). But single men far outnumbered single women (thirty six men versus eleven women). And only men left families behind to travel to Los Angeles for a cure.[86] It is likely that the gender ratio was even more imbalanced during the earlier period, when traveling alone was much less acceptable for women.

Not surprisingly, most female health seekers who appear in late nineteenth- and early twentieth-century documents were married. Writing to his mother from a Los Angeles boarding house in 1886, Charles Willard noted that a "young married lady" was "dying of consumption" in the room above his and that her husband was with her.[87] Among the "very kindly people" Martha Shaw met through her waitress job were "Mr. and Mrs. Bateman," who had "traveled around the World, for her health," and "Mr. and Mrs. Henderson," "*he* a

Lawyer and a great strong man, *she* a little woman, an invalid."[88] Carrie Pottenger, another consumptive, arrived in Southern California in 1895 with her husband, Francis Marion Pottenger (later a prominent tuberculosis physician).[89] Women without husbands occasionally came with other family members. Emma Campbell Norwood was a divorced mother of four children ages six to thirteen when tuberculosis struck in 1880. Her mother left the farm she had recently bought in Nevada to accompany her daughter and grandchildren to Burbank.[90]

Although westward travel was the preeminent recommendation for tuberculosis sufferers, it was one men could follow far more easily than women. The great majority of married women could depart for California only if their husbands were willing and able to accompany them. Most single women stayed home.

One way large numbers of women participated in health travel was as caregivers. Extolling the virtues of independence, late nineteenth-century male health seekers often described themselves as solitary adventurers. George Weeks abandoned his wife and children to embark for Southern California; he did not summon them until he was well enough to care for them. Although Charles Willard occasionally expressed gratitude for the care rendered by his wife, May, he also trivialized it by describing her services as a natural extension of her character, not real work demanding knowledge and skill. And he took credit for making the essential contribution to the household; May's services, he claimed, were important only insofar as they sustained the family breadwinner.[91]

Fortunately, some caregivers left their own accounts. Two arrived during the same period. Martha Shaw's diary emphasized her own emotions and activities, not those of her husband. Lucy Sprague's 1953 autobiography included a lengthy description of her experiences nursing her consumptive father in Southern California in 1894 and 1895.[92] (As Lucy Sprague Mitchell, she later became a famous educator.)

The two women occupied very different social positions. Lucy's father, Otho Sprague, had made a fortune in the wholesale grocery business and was one of the wealthiest men in Chicago. In Southern California, his friends included millionaire Edward L. Doheny, the discoverer of L.A. oil.[93] The family home was in the Sierra Madre foothills, approximately three miles from the city. The most famous of Southern California's health resorts, Sierra Madre was also among the most beautiful, offering panoramic mountain views.[94] Servants relieved Lucy of the most onerous housekeeping tasks. A "faithful" Swedish couple accompanied the family to Southern California; "sometimes" they also employed a cook.[95] After several months of providing care, Lucy began to attend the exclusive Marlboro School, boarding there Monday through Friday

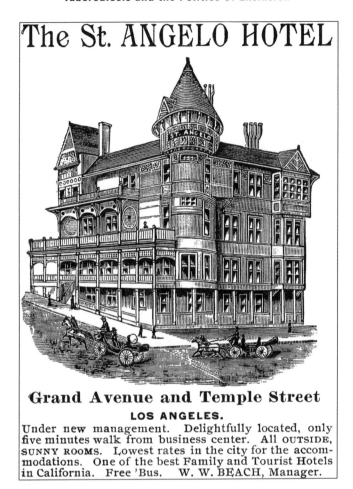

Figure 1.   Hotel where Martha Shaw worked as a waitress
Courtesy of *The Land of Sunshine*, v. 1, no. 1 (June 1894).

and returning home only for weekends. In 1896 she departed for Radcliffe College and in 1903 for the University of California at Berkeley.[96]

The Shaws, by contrast, barely could afford their cold flat in downtown Los Angeles. Although Martha received some aid from neighbors and friends, she could not shift responsibilities to servants. Instead, she assumed a double burden, working as a waitress at the St. Angelo Hotel during the day and cooking, cleaning, and providing care at night. When she left Southern California, it was to return to Topeka with her dying husband; there she nursed him another three months.

Nevertheless, some aspects of the two caregiving experiences are remarkably similar. Both Martha and Lucy were young women who arrived in Southern

California within months of sustaining devastating losses. (Martha was twenty five and Lucy just fifteen.) In January 1892, Martha had given birth to Inez, whom she proclaimed "the *sweetest, dearest, cutest, blessedest* baby ever a mother had."[97] But during the spring Inez began to cough and become fretful, and in early June the doctor diagnosed "Brain-fever." After the baby's death at the end of the month, Martha poured out her anguish in the pages of her journal. "Oh! The emptiness of my arms, the loneliness of my heart. Oh! God, ease this terrible heart-ache," she wrote at the end of June.[98] An entry on July 17 read, "I am so weary of heart I could die. I do not see how I can ever live without my Babe."[99] The sight of other babies would revive her bitter grief throughout her stay in Los Angeles. In August 1893, Lucy was traveling with her brother, Otho, whom she loved "better than anyone else," when he contracted typhoid. After their return to Chicago, he developed meningitis and died on August 18.[100]

The two women used similar language to explain their motivations to care. "No one wants me to go away with him," Martha wrote about Johnny three weeks before leaving for Los Angeles, "But if *he* insists on going, I feel it my duty to go with him; no one else would look after his welfare as I would."[101] Lucy later commented, "As a dutiful daughter, I simply did my job . . . I accepted the standards of the times that daughters belong to their families."[102]

The two women also shared a sense of banishment. Both referred to the same biblical phrase ("strangers in a strange land") their contemporaries used to describe dying consumptives in cheap lodging houses. Lucy entitled one chapter of her autobiography "My Three Years of Exile in Southern California" and described the mountains towering over her house as her only "friends in a friendless world."[103] "Good-bye to everybody," Martha wrote a few days before her departure.[104] The following week, she felt adrift in a new land. "Christmas Day, and what a mockery it is," she wrote. "Strangers, in a strange land, among strangers, more than a thousand miles from home, is not very conducive to a happy Christmas."[105] On New Year's Day, 1893, she commented, "Johnny and I went for a walk after dinner, but how could it be pleasant, when you know not a soul to say 'Howdy-do' to."[106]

The relationship to the care recipient sharpened each woman's sense of loneliness and isolation. Lucy described her father as an arrogant and selfish man who stifled his wife's creativity and was cruel to his children. When he opposed the workers in the 1894 Pullman strike, Lucy "grasped the appalling truth that Father's own business interests dominated his attitude toward people: he judged people by the amount of money they had."[107] As a sick man he made unreasonable demands. Despite his wealth, he "refused to have a nurse."[108] Because he insisted on obedience to a rigid and arbitrary schedule, he controlled "nearly every hour of every day." His daily drink had to be made in a specific way and presented "at the appointed time." On the rare occasions when Lucy was "a few minutes late, he never reproved me in words. Just took out his big watch that struck the hour, then quarters and remaining minutes and looked at it with a patient smile."[109]

Although Johnny Shaw commanded little respect in the outside world, Martha portrayed him as a tyrant at home, verbally abusing her after a miscarriage and insisting on making all household decisions. Illness appears to have aggravated his irritability and impatience. Shortly after he first became sick, she remarked, "He got so very angry at me this eve and cursed me so hard, and was so mad he wouldn't take his medicine, because he thought I took more time than I needed, to eat a lunch."[110] The following day she wrote, "He hardly lets me take time to breathe."[111] In Los Angeles she complained, "This evening I called in at Mrs. Pearson's to see their new baby and was not gone long enough to make a decent Call, yet when I came back Johnny cursed and abused me, for 'staying.' They are only across the hall from us and I was gone about 15 minutes. Oh! If I *might ever* have a kind word from Johnny."[112]

Caregiving exacted serious physical costs, too. In Sierra Madre, Lucy dreamed for the first time about her "poor old white horse." He "looked as if no one had ever loved him. He was always climbing a hill. He was always tired, with drooping head and stumbling feet. . . . Behind him moved a dim figure with a pitchfork. Whenever the old horse faltered, this pitchfork pricked his hind quarters and the old horse jerked forward at a faster pace." Although Lucy could never be certain "what this old horse symbolized," she continued to see him "at intervals" throughout her life and gradually recognized him "as a convenient barometer of fatigue."[113] "I'm almost worn out," Martha wrote on April 30, "with so much walking and my sleep and rest broken at night, by Johnny's continual coughing: it's terrible."[114] On May 23 she reported that she had "lost ten pounds, since coming here" and on June 3 that she grew "thinner every day."[115]

Both women also feared contamination. One historian notes that after Koch's discovery of the tubercle bacillus in 1882, "educated Americans slowly began to reckon with the fact that proximity to a person with tuberculosis could be dangerous. . . . This perception spread slowly and unevenly among the population during the next decade; but over time the implications of the findings were unmistakable and eventually bred a fear of associating with persons who had tuberculosis."[116] Because patients and their families were some of the first to hear the news, it is unsurprising that both Martha and Lucy had some awareness of the risk of infection. Lucy later recalled her morning ritual: "I began to empty the cuspidors. Every room except mine had at last one cuspidor partly filled with water. . . . I knew cleaning the cuspidors was dangerous work."[117] Martha wrote that although her waitress job was "hard," it was also a "blessing, in that I do not have to be so much with Johnny and run the risk of taking consumption, for he coughs dreadfully."[118]

There were some consolations. Both women derived comfort from the beauty of their new surroundings. Lucy "forgot" her "responsibilities" in hikes up Mount Wilson. "I loved the way the valley grew bigger and bigger the higher I climbed," she recalled. "I felt myself extending as my vision grew. Sometimes the valley grass was tawny, sometimes bright green with great splotches of yellow mustard and orange California poppies. Always it was beautiful; always it stretched out one's thoughts." She "missed the clouds" but loved the "fog that drifted across the valley and crept up our hill until we were surrounded with soft whiteness."[119] Although Martha insisted she preferred sunflowers to calla lilies, snow to rain, and the flatness of the prairies to the hilliness of Los Angeles, she shared Johnny's delight in the splendor around them.[120]

Success in hiding resentment conferred pride in both cases. "My heart feels like a 'chunk of lead' tonight," Martha wrote in December. "But to Johnny I am all sunshine. I thank God for the strength of will, that helps me to keep my heart ache to myself. My closest friends would never guess my unhappiness."[121] Lucy had long described herself as "conforming outwardly" to her father but "rejecting inwardly."[122] In Sierra Madre she viewed herself as a "tireless, silently suffering martyr," in a biographer's words. [123]

Although we can only wonder if either woman concealed her anger as effectively as she imagined, some evidence indicates that both exaggerated their travails. Despite the servants who lighted Lucy's load, she described herself as a "slave."[124] Her period of full-time caregiving lasted half as long as she claimed (six months as opposed to one year). Although she wrote of shouldering her burdens alone, her sister Mary was with her much of the time.[125] And she remembered her visits from Berkeley "as being more frequent and lengthy than they actually were."[126]

Martha overstated her problems by casting herself as a romantic heroine. A reader of popular women's fiction, she drew on that genre to construct her account of her life, writing in what we now would consider an excessively florid style and dramatizing her troubles. One July 20 she described herself as "away here among strangers, working and sacrificing to make a living."[127] By that date, however, she, like Johnny, had created a large circle of friends with whom she went on various jaunts. A week later, when she quit her job to nurse Johnny full time, she was able to rely on his friends as well as hers to alleviate her loneliness and furnish practical assistance.

Finally, we can ask what each woman gained from accentuating her misery. Lucy's entire autobiography was a narrative of transformation, from the obedient daughter ensnared in the ideology of her time to a famous professional woman who had successfully rebelled against her father's values.[128] By describing her father in unremittingly negative terms and exaggerating the burdens imposed on her, she emphasized the distance she had traveled.

Martha's self-portrait served a different function. Nineteenth-century American women, one literary scholar writes, "simply could not assume a stance of open rebellion against the conditions of their lives for they lacked the material means of escape or opposition. They had to stay put and submit. And so the domestic novelists made that necessity the basis on which to build a power structure of their own. Instead of rejecting the culture's value system outright, they appropriated it for their own use, subjecting the beliefs and customs that had molded them to a series of transformations that allowed them both to fulfill and transcend their appointed roles."[129] Self-pity justified at least one small act of rebellion on Martha's part. On May 30 she "went to town and bought a *nice Guitar, in a Pawn-shop, for $5.00*, some of my *tip-money* and why not, Johnny buys whiskey with my wages."[130] Even more, self-abnegation gave her a sense of moral ascendance. Her ability to submit to Johnny's will was her test, the challenge she had to face with courage and cheerfulness. From that perspective, her narrative was as much a story of triumph over adversity as Week's account of overcoming his physical weakness and frailty.

Although the journal of Margaret Love Stone is far more fragmentary than the accounts of Martha and Lucy, it enables us to glimpse another variant of the Southern California caregiving experience.[131] Born in 1847, Margaret graduated from the Steubenville Female Seminary in Steubenville, Ohio, in 1868. Three years later, she married George Stone, a merchant, and moved to his home in Erie, Pennsylvania. Their six children were born between 1875 and 1892. George survived serious abdominal surgery in 1901 but remained an invalid for the rest of his life; he sold his store in 1903 and died in 1908.[132]

The only child absent from his deathbed was the second youngest, twenty two-year-old Georgia, then seeking a cure for tuberculosis in the Pennsylvania mountains. She soon moved to Saranac Lake, New York.[133] When she still failed to improve, she decided to try her luck in the West. In 1910, Margaret accompanied Georgia to Phoenix, Arizona, and in 1911 they arrived in Los Angeles, staying first in an apartment downtown and then moving to the town of Monrovia, in the foothills of the San Gabriel Mountains.

Like Martha and Lucy twenty years before her, Margaret initially experienced her stay in Southern California as a terrible uprooting. She pined for the

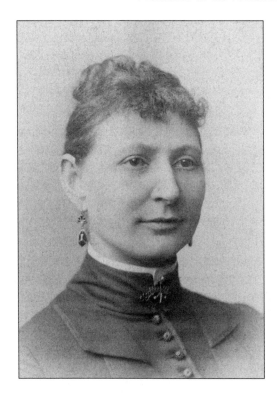

Figure 2. Margaret Love
Stone at the time of her
marriage
Courtesy of Cathryn Griffith.

five children she had left behind, as well as for her many other family members
and friends. Although the new scenery and vegetation often thrilled her, she
longed for the familiar. After buying "a box of grapes, two of peaches, and one
of quinces," for example, she commented, "I often wish for Pennsylvania fruit.
It is more tart and juicy."[134]

Because the world of tuberculosis had changed dramatically since the mid-
1890s, Margaret also faced a new set of issues. One was the growing popular
awareness of the communicable nature of the disease. Although both Martha and
Lucy had understood the dangers they faced as caregivers, they did not have to
contend with widespread fear of their care recipients. By the time Margaret
arrived in Los Angeles, however, broad-based educational programs had brought
the news about germs to a much larger public. Dr. Francis Marion Pottenger, a
prominent local advocate, argued that such programs served to counter the irrational fear of tuberculosis in the metropolis, but it is equally likely that they
accomplished the opposite.[135] Spreading the message that contact with a tubercular could be deadly, health educators transformed sufferers into menaces.

The relationship between people with TB and their doctors had also changed
dramatically since the 1890s. The physicians who dispatched patients to the West

throughout the nineteenth century had assumed they could live without strict medical supervision. Both Johnny Shaw and Otho Sprague appear to have made major treatment decisions on their own. But growing numbers of tuberculosis doctors had begun to follow Peter Dettweiler, a German doctor whose ideas were introduced to America by Paul Kretzchmar. "The smallest details of the patient's life," Kretzchmar wrote, should be "controlled by the supervising physician and nothing of any importance . . . left to his or her judgment."[136]

Such beliefs helped to spur the rise of sanatoriums, confining tuberculosis patients and subjecting them to strict regulation. In 1925, there were 536 U.S. sanatoriums, with a total of 673,338 beds.[137] The first and for many years the most famous was the Adirondack Cottage Sanitarium (later renamed Trudeau Sanitarium) at Saranac Lake. Although Margaret tells us little about Georgia's Saranac experience, it is likely that she stayed in one of the many cottages in the surrounding community. Most were basically family homes that had received only slight modification.[138] By 1920, they accommodated 1,500 patients.[139]

The Saranac model must have shaped a critical decision Margaret made shortly after arriving in Southern California. "In shifting scenes of life," she wrote at the end of 1911, "Georgia and I are out in Monrovia, California, at the foothills of Mt. Wilson. . . . We have rented a lovely furnished bungalow here, and have turned it into a small sanitarium, able to take in four patients."[140] Incorporated as a separate city in Los Angeles County in 1886, Monrovia would have been well known to Margaret as the home of the Pottenger Sanatorium, established by Dr. Pottenger in 1903. Although various small sanatoriums had begun to dot the Southern California landscape during the late nineteenth century, this was the first major facility in the area, housing an average of hundred patients.[141] In his autobiography, Pottenger wrote that he and his wife were "both exalted and depressed" by their "first sight of Monrovia." Although "the setting at the foot of the mountains was beautiful beyond words," the "lawns were parched, the streets miserably dusty, and the empty boom buildings had ceased to glitter." Nevertheless, "the beautiful surroundings, the healthful sunshine, and the tonic atmosphere won out over the disadvantages."[142] After his wife's death in 1898, Pottenger decided to become a tuberculosis specialist, traveling repeatedly to Europe to learn the latest medical knowledge.

News of Pottenger's intention to establish a sanatorium provoked what he dubbed "an epidemic fear of tuberculosis." Monrovians "considered such an institution as I proposed a personal menace, a community danger that would utterly ruin the city. Who would want to establish a home or business in a 'town of T.B.'s?'"[143] Pottenger was able to "quiet their fears" only by arguing that by isolating dangerous patients and placing them under "proper control,"

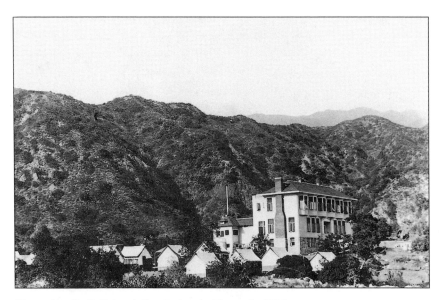

Figure 3. Dr. Pottenger's Sanatorium in Monrovia, 1920
Courtesy of Photograph Collection, Los Angeles Public Library.

the sanatorium, "would be a protection to the town rather than a source of danger." Margaret may have been aware of that history when she lost her lease on her bungalow and moved to another in January 1913. She reported with relief that they had encountered "no opposition from the neighbors to our taking ill people."[144] Perhaps the ten-year example of Pottenger's sanatorium had helped to convince the local citizenry of the strength of his arguments. In addition, of course, Margaret's facility was much smaller and the focus of little publicity.

The alarm about tuberculosis, however, probably increased the attractiveness of her tiny institution to potential clients. Times had changed greatly since the 1890s, when boarding houses and hotels had welcomed health seekers. Even the prestigious Hotel del Coronado in San Diego had advertised itself as an "ideal home" for "tourists and invalids . . . in search of health, pleasure, or comfort."[145] But after the turn of the century, TB sufferers increasingly met housing discrimination in Los Angeles, as elsewhere in the country. When Mrs. Rothstein applied for assistance from the Los Angeles Ladies and Hebrew Benevolent Society (later the Jewish Social Service Bureau) in October 1904, charity workers reported that her husband was "ill with consumption" and that, "owing to the husband's disease, accommodation was refused wherever applied for."[146] More affluent health seekers faced similar hostility. As a young man with tuberculosis in the 1880s and early 1890s, Charles Dwight Willard had experienced no trouble finding suitable accommodation in Los Angeles and Santa Barbara. But when fire destroyed his home in December 1910, he discovered that "everybody slams the door in the face of the consumptive now."[147] He asked his sister to imagine "what a soul-absorbing thing it is for a man as sick and feeble and dependent as I am to be burned out of house and home, in a country where a consumptive is treated like a leper, with every hotel, boarding house and home for rent closed against him."[148] In such a situation, Margaret's bungalow must have seemed like a particularly welcome refuge.

Local doctors appear to have sent most patients to the tiny facility and continued to provide medical care throughout their stays. Margaret's primary contact at the Pottenger Sanatorium was Dr. Frank Neall Robinson, the assistant medical director.[149] Shortly before his death, she wrote that he had been "such a wonderful physician, friend, and advisor."[150]

In opening her facility, Margaret drew not only on the example of the cottages encircling the Saranac sanatorium but also on two long-standing female traditions. One was the practice of earning extra money by taking in boarders. A historian notes that "boarding and lodging so pervaded American family life (along with the presence of servants and live-in relatives) that throughout the nineteenth century and early twentieth century, use of the term 'single-family house' is misleading."[151] Women had the primary responsibility for providing meals, cleaning the rooms, and generally watching over boarders' lives.[152]

Because Margaret furnished nursing care along with household services, she also followed the example of the countless contemporary women who parlayed healing abilities into employment. Widowhood provided, in one historian's words, "an important, if cruel, pathway into nursing. With no need for formal credentials, a woman could offer her experience of caring for a dying husband as her qualification to nurse."[153] Because Margaret's husband had been ill for seven years, she may have felt especially competent to nurse others. And since his death, she had received ample experience delivering tuberculosis care.

Running a "sanitarium" proved more onerous than she had anticipated. In 1911, she was sixty-four and suffered from numerous ailments. African American servants did the gardening and some of the heavy housework. Margaret's youngest daughter, Dorothy, who joined the household in September 1912, furnished other assistance. But servants often left abruptly, and Dorothy was soon swept up in the Monrovia social life, entertaining various beaux and participating in the town's May spring carnival. In July 1913, Margaret complained about "the never ending housekeeping."[154] When Dorothy took a short vacation a few months later, Margaret found herself "overwhelmed with work." "I am so tired through my hips," she continued, "and ache with a feeling that I cannot keep on my feet."[155] The following year her daily round aggravated her knee and back problems. "I was up at seven," she wrote in 1914, "and took care of the chickens before breakfast and worked around more freely than I've been able to do for weeks." By the afternoon, however, her knee was "so very lame."[156] Four days later she wrote, "I started out with my duties this morning thinking my sciatica was much improved, but, before breakfast was ready, I found the pain acute, and all day it has pained me though I have performed a number of duties."[157] Still feeling "great discomfort" at the end of the month, she commented, "I must wonder sometimes if I am going to fail in strength." By October, doctors had begun to warn about the need for surgery. "Oh!" she wrote, "To feel well again, full of vigor, to accomplish my work with ease."[158]

Nursing services further taxed her strength. Private-duty nurses provided some care to the sickest patients. After the first nursing schools opened in 1873, such nurses increasingly became available. Beginning in 1905, many were trained specifically to care for tuberculosis patients.[159] But the presence of nurses had costs as well as benefits for Margaret. "Mrs Glacer," for example, "was rather nice but did not want to be told to do as I suggested, though it was seldom that I meddled. Really, a few times I positively disliked her though I tried to think we were thankful to have her."[160] And private duty nurses were not always available. "Two patients very ill," Margaret noted in November 1914, "and it's lots of care on us."[161]

Caregiving also imposed emotional distress. In July 1913, Margaret commented, "About midnight Dorothy discovered that one of the patients, Mrs. B., had taken strychnine to commit suicide. . . . Dorothy was awfully nervously wrought up over it."[162] The plights of other patients had particular resonance for Margaret. We can well imagine her grim sense of foreboding as she watched the relentless deterioration of a young man close in age to Georgia. "Our patients are gaining," Margaret reported in September 1913, "all but Mr. McLaren, who is in bed again with temperature. I am so sorry for him—only 22 yrs. old—eldest child of a Presbyterian minister who has his own way to make and had a good start at it. He came here not really sure he was a T.B. and hoped in six months to be home at his work, cured. For a time it seemed as if he would be, but for several months he has only lost."[163] Care for the paying patients also occasionally clashed with the needs of Margaret's sick daughter. "Georgia is not well," Margaret wrote the same month, "and we think some of going away together. To get some one to fill our duties here (there's the rub)."[164] The conflict between public and private responsibilities must have been especially intense when Georgia's condition drastically declined at the end of the year. "We had a nice Christmas day here," Margaret reported on New Year's Eve, "but since then Georgia has been taken ill."[165] Although Martha wrote little in the diary the following spring, there was an entry for May 31, 1914: "Georgia, dear child, has been in bed since Easter and from Christmas until along in March."[166] After her death, on July 17, 1914, Margaret continued to operate the facility for another year. Now every dying patient must have forced her to relive her own painful loss.

Nevertheless, Margaret had at least some ways to remain emotionally distant. Although she welcomed both Japanese and Jewish patients, they remained "the other." She described the Japanese as "intelligent" but also referred to them as "Japs."[167] Soon after noting that Mr. Green was "quite a companion of all of us, a comrade of Georgia's in the forenoons and jollying Dorothy in the afternoons,"[168] Margaret fretted: "He and Dorothy are most too congenial—he a Jew and a pleasant one at that."[169] Margaret had harsher words for another Jewish patient. Mr. Katz "was cross and hard to please. He is difficult at the best of times."[170] Other patients also occasionally offended. A devout Christian, she was horrified when her first group of patients violated the Sabbath. And she never forgot that her primary relationship to all patients was financial. One of her most arduous tasks was collecting money. One patient departed "owing us $130" at a time when another was "back $45."[171] There also was constant anxiety about filling the beds. "Dorothy and I have come to an unexpected, anxious place," Margaret noted in the middle of April 1915. "In a little over a week, all our patients will have gone. . . . . People, though ill, do not have the money, and our expenses are very high."[172]

Growing fears about germs created other problems. Although the neighbors had not prevented Margaret from caring for sick people, she knew she often would have to conceal the nature of their disease. After a second visit from one of Dorothy's beaux, Margaret wrote, "Dorothy was so nervous when he was here before, because she thought if he knew there were TB's here, he would never come back."[173] When a cousin from the East "only stayed a little while" at the house, Margaret scoffed, "Really, she acted afraid of T.B."[174] But Margaret had her own anxieties, especially for Dorothy. In August 1915, Margaret wrote, "Dorothy had her lungs examined today by Dr. Kirschner, and he declared them sound. I am going around so glad and thankful. I look forward to these examinations with dread. She has had several."[175]

Margaret may have been especially "glad and thankful" because she knew that might be one of the last examinations Dorothy would be forced to undergo. They were now "getting ready to evacuate this home."[176] Dorothy was engaged to be married, and Margaret had sold the facility to Dr. Kirschner, who operated several "cottages for the treatment of tuberculosis" in Monrovia.[177] After Dorothy's September wedding, Margaret returned to Erie to live with one of her older daughters. In September 1926, she was back in Monrovia, now living with Dorothy and her family. She died in July 1928.[178]

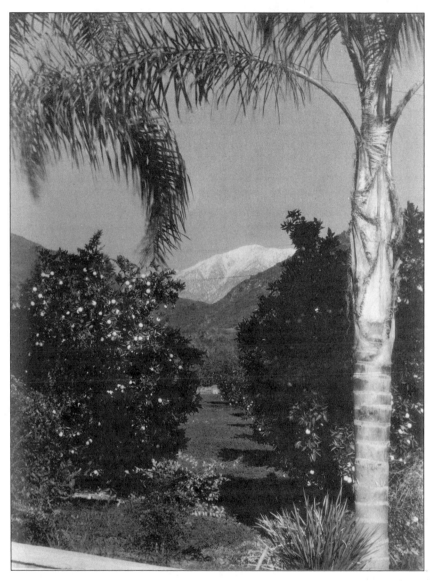

Figure 4. 1920 Ad for Los Angeles. The title read: "California sunshine shines on these groves the year round, filling the oranges with sunshine and health"

Courtesy of the University of Southern California, on behalf of the USC Specialized Libraries and Archival Collections.

Returning to Southern California in the 1920s, Margaret must have noticed many changes. That decade's great boom transformed both the metropolis and the booster industry that sustained it. The city population jumped from 57,000 to 1.24 million, more than 100 percent.[179] The county (which included, in addition to Los Angeles City, several small cities and large unincorporated areas) grew even more rapidly, from 936,455 to nearly 2.25 million, a 135 percent increase.[180] Although large areas of the county remained agricultural, suburbs, manufacturing plants, and freeways covered more and more land. The recently established motion picture industry attracted growing numbers of actors and writers, who made Los Angeles the movie capital of the world.[181]

In 1921, local businessmen organized the All-Year Club, which gradually surpassed the Chamber of Commerce as the city's leading booster organization. The impetus came from a landlord's complaint to a prominent journalist that tourism flourished only during the winter months. As its name implies, the new group sought to convince easterners and midwesterners that Los Angeles offered manifold delights to vacationers throughout the year and that its summers were as pleasant as its winters.[182]

One observer notes that Los Angeles traditionally has been marketed simultaneously "as a tranquilizer and as a stimulant."[183] Even while flooding the rest of the county with information about the glamor of Hollywood, promoters trumpeted the city's salubrious climate, restful beaches, and restorative mountains.[184] The giant citrus industry further cemented the connection between Los Angeles and health. Capitalizing on the 1915 discovery of vitamin C, Sunkist launched a massive advertising campaign focused on the therapeutic powers of the vaunted fruit of the land.[185]

But boosters no longer directed their appeal toward consumptives. As confidence in the climate cure waned, eastern doctors urged patients to place themselves under strict medical supervision at home rather than purchasing tickets to the West. Gradually, Southern California withdrew its welcome. Although large numbers of health seekers continued to arrive, public health authorities and private charities actively sought to retard the influx.

Chapter 2

Strategies of Exclusion

As the new century opened, the booster enterprise increasingly met opposition. The primary critics were public health officials, who argued that the welfare of Los Angeles required exclusion, not unlimited expansion, and proposed various measures to seal the borders. Growing concerns about germs bolstered the public health campaign. In California, as in the rest of the nation, health officials and advocates launched a massive educational campaign in the 1890s. A broad array of films, posters, exhibits, and lectures gradually convinced the public that tuberculosis was a communicable, not a hereditary, disease and that even casual contact with sufferers could be dangerous.[1] As a result, Los Angelenos no longer regarded health seekers as ideal visitors or neighbors.

The growing focus on germs also strengthened the tendency to blame foreigners for disease. As a political scientist writes, "The imagery from infectious disease suggests an outside agent that invades the body and causes illness."[2] Californians had special reason for accusing outsiders of introducing tuberculosis. After noting that TB caused "one in every seven deaths" in California, the State Board of Health declared in 1908 that "the high death rate" was "not normal to the state" and that "consumption should be a rare disease." The fault lay with the "many" people "coming here from other states, seeking the advantages of our climate, but seeking it too late."[3]

Two years later, the board published data to buttress the claim that a high tuberculosis mortality rate was "not normal" to California. Of the people who had died of the disease the previous year, "only" 30.2 percent "were natives of the State, having been here for life." The "per cent born elsewhere, but who were residents of 10 years' standing, was 24.5 for 1909."[4] The obvious conclusion was that the disease was an "imported infection."[5] Those figures, of course, are basically meaningless because the Los Angeles population as a whole doubled during the 1890s and tripled during the 1900s.[6] Long-term residents thus accounted for relatively few deaths from any cause in 1909. Despite that problem, the board issued similar statistics year after year and used them as the basis for urging the legislature to defend the state against consumptives from the East.

The policy of exclusion also stemmed from beliefs about other characteristics of the affected population. Although nineteenth-century experts had assumed that tuberculosis struck all segments of society equally, turn-of-the-century authorities throughout the United States increasingly identified the disease with subordinate groups. The State Board of Health declared that California was "deluged at certain seasons of the year with patients, many too . . . poor to return home."[7] Statistics again seemed to offer support. A particularly important "fact" was that "seventy-five per cent of the patients dying of tuberculosis" in the state had "family incomes less than one thousand dollars."[8]

Because people with weakened resistance as a result of stress, poverty, poor nutrition, and repeated exposure in overcrowded dwellings are most likely to contract tuberculosis, we can assume that low-income families experienced unusually high rates of the disease. Nevertheless, the board's new "fact," like the claim that outsiders brought the disease to California, is open to challenge. The diagnosis of tuberculosis remained inexact throughout the early twentieth century.[9] Moreover, although a 1907 California law required physicians to report tuberculosis,[10] compliance was far from perfect, especially in the early years. Some doctors may simply have been negligent; some may have resented any official incursions into their autonomy; and some may have succumbed to the pressure of patients who wanted to conceal the disease to avoid the stigma surrounding it.[11] Death certificates tended to provide more accurate information, but mortality data, too, may have exaggerated the proportion of poor cases. Many life insurance companies denied benefits to families in cases of tuberculosis, and it therefore is likely that some physicians recorded other causes of death in deference to the wishes of survivors.[12] Patients who were too poor to consult private physicians or purchase life insurance may have been especially likely to be labeled tubercular in official reports.

Anxieties about contagion meshed with and intensified fears about poor people. Even before news about germs spread throughout society, late nineteenth-century commentators in Los Angeles had defined indigent consumptives as threatening by associating them with tramps. The new bacteriological knowledge bred fresh worries. A recurrent theme in the writings of early twentieth century health officials was the failure of germs to respect class barriers. "There is no doubt," the Board of Health wrote in 1906, that many people who died of tuberculosis during the past year "contracted the disease from cases coming here without the means for proper care." Those "infected strangers, living in dark and ill-ventilated rooms, eating at cheap restaurants and expectorating everywhere, will infect more natives than ten times the number who reside in good homes where care is exercised."[13] The contrast between the strangers who expectorated "everywhere" and the residents of "good homes" who took "care" reminds us that the practices of indigent health seekers were considered as important as the conditions in which they slept and ate. Most doctors believed that sputum (the phlegm coughed up by infected lungs) was the major source of tubercle bacilli and that poor people were especially likely to spread disease because they expectorated wherever they wished.[14] Some observers added that the poor failed to comply with public health advice because they were "vicious" as well as "ignorant."[15]

But worries about germs were not the only cause of the increased hostility and suspicion surrounding poor people with tuberculosis. The progressive movement of the late nineteenth and early twentieth centuries placed a high premium on economic efficiency, and consumptives represented a high proportion of charity recipients. In a discussion of "the indigent consumptive" in the Southwest, Ernest A. Sweet, a former surgeon in the U.S. Public Health Service, concluded, "It is not alone because he is a sufferer from tuberculosis that he is unwelcome, but because he is a pauper as well."[16] Concerns about the economic burdens imposed by poor people with tuberculosis soon would dominate public policy in California as well as in the rest of the nation.

The virulence of the rhetoric about poor consumptives also arose from the belief that they suffered disproportionately from advanced disease. The same combination of personal traits and external conditions that appeared to increase their vulnerability to contracting tuberculosis was assumed to diminish their ability to fight it.[17] Like such recovered health seekers as George F. Weeks, many early twentieth century observers emphasized the negative traits of the very sick. Conspicuous symptoms were singled out for disgust. Dr. Sweet declared, "The far advanced consumptives . . . are objectionable, those who present no appearance of invalidism being in an entirely different category from those who exhibit every evidence of the ravages of the disease."[18] A physician writing in the *Southern California Practitioner* alerted his colleagues to the special dangers posed by consumptives who were "palpably stricken with death."[19] Fear of contagion, of course, made the signs of tuberculosis especially distasteful. But symptoms had meaning even apart from the communicability they betrayed. By the turn of the century, emaciation, the most visible "ravage" of tuberculosis, must have seemed particularly repugnant. The new kind of masculinity then emerging valorized physical bulk, not the wiry leanness that previously had been the ideal.[20]

Advanced disease also declared itself in sounds. As Susan Sontag writes, the "prototypical TB symptom" was coughing: "The sufferer is wracked by coughs, then sinks back, recovers breath, breathes normally; then coughs again."[21] Pasadena residents who signed petitions urging the Los Angeles County Board of Supervisors to close a health camp for indigent patients in 1909 argued not only that they represented a "menace" but also that "the coughing of the patients is constant night and day, and while we have every sympathy with the victims of the disease we do not think it fair or right to be compelled to hear their distressing coughing day and night continuously."[22] In addition to producing offensive noises, persistent coughing indicated that bodies were out of control at a time when order and predictability were highly valued.

And advanced disease exacerbated the other problems associated with the poor. Because the sputum of people in the last states of disease was especially dangerous,[23] they had the greatest potential to harm the rest of the population. But poor people were assumed to be extremely careless about safeguarding the health of others. Very sick patients who were poor also inflicted the greatest economic costs, relying on financial assistance programs and free medical care for months and occasionally years. Conflating medical and social characteristics, health authorities throughout the United States expressed unusual antipathy toward poor people with advanced tuberculosis. Herman M. Biggs, the chief medical officer of the New York City Department of Health, tried to reserve places at his flagship sanatorium for people with "incipient" cases who could be "restor[ed] to permanent usefulness in the community."[24] As his biographer explained, Biggs believed that "there were individuals . . . whose lives were so worthless to the community that it would be an unpardonable waste of public funds to give them the benefit of sanatorium care."[25] Viewed as pariahs, these "hopeless third state cases, chronic alcoholics, and the persistently incorrigible" found beds only in large, overcrowded, city hospitals.[26] Many California officials similarly equated productivity and social worth and relied on that value system when distributing scarce sanatorium beds.

In the West as in the East, heightened anxieties about tuberculosis found expression in the early twentieth-century drive to restrict immigration throughout the country.[27] Long before Californians began to link disease and immigration control, however, they sought to repel migrants from other states. Because elite groups assumed that poor people with tuberculosis were especially likely to spread germs, overwhelm the public purse, and suffer from advanced disease, the campaign of exclusion focused on them. The one major exception was the opening salvo, a 1900 request from the State Board of Health to the legislature to bar entry of all people with tuberculosis.[28] That proposal provoked vigorous protest. Norman Bridge, a prominent tuberculosis physician who came to Southern California to cure his own disease, pointed out that the proposed quarantine was patently impractical: "All passenger trains would have to be delayed several hours till all the passengers could be examined. The general appearance of the travelers could not be relied upon to tell who are dangerous consumptives, for some mortally sick ones look in the face very well, and nine-tenths of all tuberculous patients could easily hoodwink any inspector."[29] Other critics decried the proposal as inhumane. Dr. Francis Marion Pottenger, who had accompanied his consumptive wife to Southern California, wrote that "patients have enough to bear without being treated as lepers, and the society which would add an unnecessary stigma to them is culpable and inhumane. What one of us would want to be treated as a social outcast? We may be well today, but what have we to insure that we have not latent tuberculosis processes within our lungs that may be started into activity in the future? What one of us has not a friend or dear one who is afflicted with this disease?"

But Pottenger had another, even more important objection: "Unless the law will allow a discrimination to be made between the man with the money and the man without, then such a measure can not stand."[30] He later wrote that had the 1900 quarantine bill passed, "it would have deprived Southern California of a great number of men and women who were to be counted among her most valued and influential citizens, many of whom came here to seek recovery from tuberculosis for themselves or some member of their families."[31] After the bill's defeat, officials sought to impose quarantine by other means. Most measures were carefully targeted toward the poor alone.

Chastened by the opposition to its first proposal, the Board of Health emphasized strategies that would not restrict the entry of migrants with the potential to become those "most valued and influential citizens." In 1913, the board urged that railroads be required "to add a clause to the printed conditions on each overland ticket which every passenger signs, to the effect that before a ticket is issued each person suffering with tuberculosis must obtain and file with the railway company a permit from the State Board of Health having juris-diction over the point of destination, or file in duplicate a statement that he is provided with sufficient funds to provide proper care for himself while away."[32] Two years later, Edythe Tate-Thompson, the newly appointed director of the board's Bureau of Tuberculosis, posted warnings in East Coast railroad stations, clinics, and employment agencies, stating that California had no free beds for nonresidents and that they should come only if they had a year's financial support.[33]

At the behest of the Board of Health, California congressmen introduced the 1916 Kent Bill stipulating that nonresident tubercular people would either be sent to their homes or supported in part by the federal government. As the secretary of the board remarked, one of the primary goals was to "discourage migration."[34] Both the board and local TB advocates campaigned vigorously for the bill, flooding Congress, the surgeon general, and even President Wilson with information.[35] Tate-Thompson circulated a newsletter noting, "A large proportion of the migrating tuberculosis cases arrive at their destination with limited funds, which are soon totally exhausted, the burden of their care falling upon the local community. In the Los Angeles County Hospital, during a single year, but of a thousand cases of tuberculosis, less than fifty were Californians." The newsletter urged support of the Kent bill, which "offers relief to the states that for years have been the dumping grounds for non-resident indigent tuberculous."[36]

In 1918, the Board of Health responded quickly and angrily to reports that the U.S. Army was furnishing cash to the many men rejected because of tuberculosis and encouraging them to travel west in search of a good climate and appropriate work. The board wrote letters to various federal officials urging that the men instead be given tickets home and dispatched Tate-Thompson to Washington to plead the case in person.[37] In December 1922, she took another tack, writing to Surgeon General Hugh S. Cummings:

> All during the Autumn and Winter we have received complaints from passengers using the Santa Fe regarding the travel of advanced cases of tuberculosis, many of whom appear to be ex-service men en route to Los Angeles, Albuquerque, and Phoenix. These patients naturally use the dining car and according to the complaints are not supplied with sputum cups and in some instances it appears that the berths occupied by these people have been resold before the car reached its destination.

Tate-Thompson asked Cummings to request the Pullman Company (which manufactured and operated the sleeping cars on U.S. railroads) not to resell the berths and to notify the U.S. Veterans Bureau that it must give the men "printed instructions and see that they are supplied with sputum cups."[38] Two years later she reported that "the advent of so many ex-service men with tuberculosis who are being sent into this state" had "brought serious problems" not only to the communities where they settled but also to "their families who have insisted upon following them." And there was the "added social problem" of "the divorced wives of these men, many of whom are ill without funds."[39]

Charitable societies provided critical support to the public health campaign. Some urged East Coast branches to discontinue the practice of encouraging poor tuberculars to travel to Southern California.[40] One of the first to comply was the New York Charity Organization Society, the city's major philanthropic society, which sent a letter to 8,600 physicians calling attention to "the consequences arising from the practice of sending poor consumptives to such states as Arizona, Colorado, and California." "Extensive experience" had demonstrated that "difficult as it may be for a poor man to recover from tuberculosis in this city, he is better off here among his friends and relatives, where there are more adequate hospital and dispensary facilities, than he is far from home, where he is thrown entirely upon his resources and where the great number of consumptives willing to work at the lowest wages make the finding of employment . . . almost impossible." Physicians thus should refrain from encouraging consumptives to depart unless they had promises of "suitable" and remunerative work or "at their disposal at least $250 in addition to railroad fare."[41]

Consumptives who applied to Los Angeles charitable organizations were provided only with train fare home. An 1898 article in the Los Angeles *Evening Express* complained about "H. Jimoniski, late of New York, formerly of Russia and a direct descendant of Abraham" who was "a little evaporated Russian with a perpetual whine and a silvery voice which sounded like a cheap phonograph with the rolls worn out." His most notable feature, however, was "his nerve," which "was something wonderful." He had "coolly informed" a local charity that he was too sick to work and needed assistance. Fortunately, that group sent him to St. Louis, where he had family.[42] The Board of Health reported a second example in 1905: "A young lady eighteen or twenty years of age, from one of the States of the Middle West, was advised to go to California, where she would speedily get rid of her troublesome cough." But "her disease progressed rapidly, and had it not been for the charity of strangers who sent her home, she would have added one more victim to the list of [those who] 'died inside one year.' "[43]

Although charitable organizations claimed that they transported only those clients who were well enough to travel, it was not easy to make accurate assessments. The March 10, 1902, case files of the Ladies and Hebrew Benevolent Society recorded the purchase of train tickets for the ailing Mr. Schwartz and his wife. The following week's report read: "Upon the day of the intended departure of the Schwartz family for Philadelphia, after reaching the depot Mr. Schwartz expired, necessary arrangements for the funeral had to be made and change of tickets attended to, as the departure of Mrs. Schwartz was delayed for two months."[44] Other clients must have died en route.

In 1909, the Los Angeles County Board of Supervisors followed the example of private charities. Invoking the principle of local responsibility for indigents, the board enacted a rule that consumptives seeking public assistance would instead by given one-way train fares out of town.[45] Four years later the Los Angeles County Department of Charities returned forty-five tubercular patients and their families; private charitable agencies transported an additional hundred.[46] In 1917, a physician at a city tuberculosis clinic noted that, with the help of that department, he had "deported back to their home town or city many tuberculars." As he explained, "It is a far cheaper method of caring for them than it is to allow them to stay in the County Hospital until they die."[47] Worries about the germs spread by traveling consumptives seem not to have been directed toward those returning home.

The emphasis on exclusion also retarded efforts to provide free or low-cost care. The first proposals to establish either a state or county sanatorium met defeat partly as a result of fears that such a facility would attract invalids from other states.[48] When the Los Angeles County Board of Supervisors announced plans to construct four new buildings for the overcrowded county hospital in 1902, the Municipal League, the major Progressive organization, protested that the proposal would involve exorbitant expense to taxpayers. In addition, the league claimed, the new buildings would serve as an "apparent invitation to indigent invalids from all over the Union to come to this country and be cared for."[49] In response, several trade unions signed petitions urging the board to proceed with the "plans for enlarging the county hospital and for making that notoriously inadequate and antiquated institution more modernized and comfortable."[50] But the league held firm, continuing to oppose any expansion until the board agreed to a compromise, reducing the number of new buildings from four to two."[51]

A similar controversy engulfed the Jewish community. The first Jews to settle in Los Angeles were Germans, many of whom quickly rose to prominence in the city's business and professional life.[52] The arrival of large numbers of east European immigrants after the turn of the century provoked horror. The major German Jewish journal, the *B'nai B'rith Messenger*, warned that "immense hordes of Jewish Immigrants" were importing "immoral and unsanitary conditions."[53] And many were sick and poor. Echoing the sentiments expressed by the gentile elite, the *Messenger* declared in 1902, "We have often dwelt upon the folly of sending penniless invalids to the West. There is room in the Pacific states for people of energy who can enter into the upbuilding of this great country with vim and vigor. But this whole country is overrun with people who have come from all parts of the world in quest of health, with little health and less means."[54] In 1912, the paper wrote, "With the advent of cold weather in the East the annual hegira of destitute consumptives to this city begins, making the lives of those who are in some way connected with the local charities most miserable." Readers should "understand that the sick poor referred to are all strangers."[55]

Not surprisingly, the Industrial Removal Office, responsible for dispersing Jewish immigrants throughout the country, received little support.[56] In 1912, the Ladies and Hebrew Benevolent Society reported, "We have had 160 applications from the Removal Office for families and single persons to be sent to Los Angeles this winter. We gave our permission to 117 and refused 43. Though we had an agreement with the Removal Office not to send sick or indigent persons, some managed to slip in."[57] Because the Panama Canal threatened to provide direct access to the West Coast from Europe, its construction sparked new worries. "The pity of it all," one observer wrote in the *Messenger*, was that the typical Jewish newcomer would be "the poor and downtrodden, the uneducated and sick of other lands."[58]

Migrants with TB found few sources of assistance. In 1906, the newly established Hebrew Consumptive Relief Association (HCRA) provided support for two Jewish patients at Barlow Sanatorium;[59] in 1913, eight patients were placed at various private facilities.[60] Dissatisfied with such paltry efforts, trade unions affiliated with the left-leaning Workmen's Circle organized a rival group, the Southern California Jewish Consumptive Relief Association (JCRA), dedicated to establishing a Jewish sanatorium open to consumptives from all parts of the county. Old settlers were aghast. "The people behind the new institution" were "treading on dangerous ground," wrote Isaac Norton, HCRA president. "We ought not to induce the sick to come here." If the JCRA insisted on establishing a new institution, it should be a small, local one, seeking funding only in Los Angeles and restricting eligibility to county residents.[61] Other critics pointed to the negative example of Denver, where the establishment of a national Jewish sanatorium had helped to attract large numbers of indigent patients.[62] As the JCRA pressed forward with its plans, opposition continued to mount. In 1914, local newspapers announced that the Los Angeles County Board of Supervisors had drafted an ordinance prohibiting the establishment in the county of any institution that had not received the consent of 75 percent of all neighbors within a one-mile radius.[63]

Seeking to repel rather than woo invalids, health officials often defined themselves in opposition to the boosters. But the similarities between the two groups were as striking as their differences. Like the publicists, health authorities defined the "right kind" of people as white and middle class and worked relentlessly to advance their interests. After the defeat of an early state quarantine bill, all exclusionary strategies were carefully targeted toward the poor alone. In addition, public health officials argued that illness was not a normal and inevitable part of life in Southern California. In their reports, as in the promotional literature, the ill represented everything Los Angelenos were supposed to be able to avoid—dependence, uncertainty, deterioration, and premature death. All advocates of services for TB sufferers would have to acknowledge those attitudes.

Chapter 3

Creating a Tuberculosis Program

The campaign to establish free and low-cost services in Los Angeles both reflected and reinforced the growing hostility surrounding poor people affected by the disease. A key argument for creating hospitals and sanatoriums was that they promoted public safety by segregating the patients most likely to spread germs.[1] But all institutions soon had long waiting lists; many people urged to accept placement either refused to do so or fled soon after arriving; and restrictive residence requirements disqualified some patients considered especially threatening. Far from increasing support for hospitals and sanatoriums, statements about the need for isolation often hardened attitudes about the indigent consumptives living in the community and undermined any sense of public responsibility for them.

The other central argument, that institutions advanced economic efficiency by transforming patients into workers, strengthened the conviction that people too sick to reenter the labor force lacked social value. After institutions opened, advocates contended that the restoration of "work force capacity" required rehabilitation programs as well as medical care because long periods of enforced idleness nourished the dependent spirit of the poor. That assertion bolstered the belief that the indigent sick were malingerers, all too willing to impose excessive burdens on others, and highlighted the high proportion of charitable assistance consumed by people with tuberculosis.

Another problem was that the two major justifications for care had practical implications that often clashed. To reduce the peril tuberculosis sufferers posed, programs had to focus on "advanced cases," who produced the most "poisonous" sputum. Programs seeking to return sick people to the labor force, however, needed to target those in early stages of disease. And regardless of which goal they emphasized, all programs were expensive. Their expansion thus provoked new complaints about the financial costs imposed by tuberculosis patients. Attempts to save money by restricting eligibility raised fears that a large, dangerous population would remain uncontrolled.

Although a few private groups founded small institutions for poor people with TB, most free and low-cost tuberculosis services were the responsibility of government agencies, including the California State Board of Health, the Los Angeles City Health Department, the Los Angeles County Department of Health, which had jurisdiction over the unincorporated areas of the county as well as several small cities within its borders, and the Los Angeles County Department of Charities, which operated both the county hospital and sanatorium. Local advocacy groups spearheaded a massive health-education campaign, provided some funding for tuberculosis care, and continually pressed the government to increase public expenditure. In 1902 physicians founded the Southern California Anti-Tuberculosis League. When that organization became the California Tuberculosis Association in 1907, doctors created the Los Angeles Tuberculosis Association (later the Los Angeles County Tuberculosis and Health Association) to continue the local work.[2] The same year, city physicians organized the Society for the Study and Prevention of Tuberculosis (soon renamed the Los Angeles Tuberculosis and Health Association).

Surveying the Los Angeles area in the early twentieth century, advocacy groups easily could see how much work remained to be done. The major facility serving the poor was Los Angeles County Hospital (later Los Angeles General Hospital), founded in 1878 east of the river on Mission Road. A physician employed at the facility during its first decade concluded "from personal observation" that the clientele consisted overwhelmingly of "the improvident foreigner and the dissipated American."[3] Because the primary function of nineteenth-century hospitals was to shelter the chronically ill, it is unsurprising that consumption was a major diagnosis. According to L.A. records, "phthsis" (an antiquated name for tuberculosis) afflicted 568 of the first 3,879 hospital patients.[4] A rare surviving case file from the turn of the century discussed a forty-two-year-old "steve moulder" from Ohio whose "present trouble" started "about 10 years ago" although he had been "up and down since then." Three months before his admission on November 19, 1899, he "began to get quite ill" and decided he had "la Grippe." He coughed a "great deal" and was "much emaciated." A "sputum examination" found "tubercle bacilli in abundance." He died in the hospital on January 11, 1900.[5]

Like other contemporary hospitals, the county facility gradually gained social legitimacy by allying with new developments in scientific medicine. In

1885, the hospital became affiliated with the newly opened College of Medicine of the University of Southern California, and faculty members began to serve as attending physicians. The first interns arrived a few years later. After the founding of the nursing school in 1895, graduates slowly replaced untrained nurses.[6]

Nevertheless, the quality of medical treatment remained dismal. In 1914, the Los Angeles Society for the Study and Prevention of Tuberculosis wrote that "the care of the unfortunate creatures who were sent to the County Hospital may have been little less than horrible in the cold-bloodedness with which they were allowed to eke out their few remaining years of life in the unsanitary ward known as 'Old Ward 10.'"[7] An 1899 account enables us to glimpse that care. In a letter to the Los Angeles County Board of Supervisors, a patient described the experiences of three consumptives on his ward. The first, "a Scotch boy," had been "brought to the hospital with hemorrhages" and died "under most pitiable circumstances." During the night "he fell out of bed in his restlessness and in so doing overturned a toilet jar half filled with urine and the vomit of undigested food. The stench . . . immediately floated throughout the ward all the rest of the night." The nurse who was called "at first . . . paid no attention to the filth but finally . . . cleaned the place in a perfunctory manner." When the boy's bed "was made filthy by the excrements from his body," the nurse wiped him with "clothes enriched with filth." A few nights before, a doctor had ordered a plaster for the boy. The nurse, however, refused to apply it until the letter-writing patient "remonstrated" with her. Another "pathetic instance of abuse on the part of the nurses" concerned a man "brought to the hospital dying of consumption." When other patients helped him sit in a chair, the nurse insisted that he return to bed unaided. A third patient "was ordered to leave the hospital . . . because he refused to work beyond his strength."[8]

After the Los Angeles County Medical Association argued in 1901 that the overcrowded tuberculosis ward subverted the goal of providing fresh air, some patients were housed in tents on the grounds.[9] But that solution did not please everyone. One man wrote to the County Board of Supervisors in January 1908 that he was "sleeping in an open, isolated tent without stove and insufficient bed covering." He asked "to live his remaining life in bearable condition."[10]

The Board of Supervisors continued to receive complaints after the opening of a new tuberculosis ward in 1910. "The new tuberculosis building is certainly a vast improvement on the old building which was used for these patients," wrote the County Medical Association, "but if this building is to really be of value during the coming summer it will be necessary to screen in the outside porches." There also was "an urgent need" for "reclining chairs." And noise, smoke, and dust filled the facility from nearby railroad yards and industries.[11]

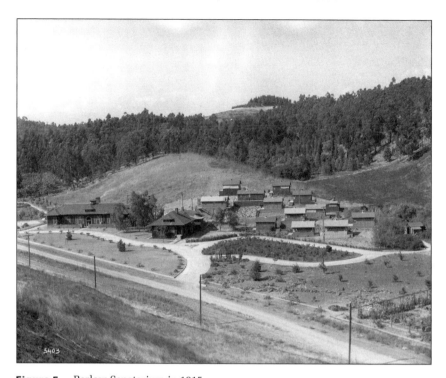

Figure 5.   Barlow Sanatorium in 1915

Courtesy of the University of Southern California, on behalf of the USC Specialized Libraries and Archival Collections.

Other observers noted that overcrowding remained a serious problem. Beds were packed tightly in the ward; many lined the corridors.[12] A state official who visited tuberculosis patients in 1921 wrote that the "overcrowding could not have been worse if half of Los Angeles had been stricken with plague."[13] A bond issue passed two years later raised funds for a new building, but that facility did not open until 1934.[14]

Advocates wanted not only to reform the county hospital but also to provide sanatorium care for tuberculosis patients. Although the first L.A. sanatoriums served affluent health seekers, advocates increasingly argued that poor people had the greatest need for the regulation those facilities imposed. The 1923 directory of the National Tuberculosis Association listed three free or low-cost private sanatoriums in the Los Angeles area.[15] Founded by Walter Jarvis Barlow, another physician who came to Southern California to recover from consumption, Barlow Sanatorium (now Barlow Respiratory Hospital) opened in 1902.[16] One historian notes that the sanatorium's "Board of Directors and the Advisory Board always would read like a social register of Southern California's top business, civic, and society leaders."[17] And, indeed, the facility served the interests of the Los Angeles elite in various ways. Strict eligibility criteria discouraged migration. "We received many letters of inquiry from invalids at some distance from the city," the resident physician wrote in 1911. "To all such treatment was refused, as the institution is kept up for the poor of Los Angeles County alone, or for those who have lived in the County at least one year."[18] In addition, the facility promoted the well-being of the entire community. Its "special work" was the "isolation of cases among the poorer classes"; as a result, "much good work" would "be done in preventing the spread of the disease."[19] After acquiring middle-class values and habits along with their cures, discharged patients were expected to "carry the gospel of right living to others."[20]

The sanatorium also affirmed two guiding principles of U.S. welfare policy—categorizing the poor and upholding the "work ethic." Unlike the county hospital filled with "dissipated" individuals, this facility restricted admission to "the worthy tuberculous poor."[21] As Barlow wrote, "The cases are taken from the poorer walks of life, yet the majority of them are refined people."[22] To enhance "feelings of self worth," patients were put to work as soon as possible, growing vegetables, planting trees, repairing cottages, and constructing concrete walks.[23]

But it was not possible to advance all goals simultaneously. Intent on transforming as many patients as possible into productive workers, the institution gave preference to "curable cases,"[24] thus leaving the most dangerous patients in the community. The resident physician acknowledged that "to isolate any considerable number of advanced cases of an infectious disease is a most valuable means of helping to eradicate the affection by protecting those who are yet unaffected." Nevertheless, he concluded that "it is even more important, from an economic standpoint, to recognize and treat the early and curable instances of such disease, in order to preserve the life of the subject and prevent the long term of invalidism that is still the rule."[25]

In the end, however, the choice of clientele was not entirely the administrators' to make. As one observer noted in 1905, "Circumstances over which the institution has had no control, have made it necessary, in a number of instances, to admit patients whose condition gave not even the faintest hope of improvement." The sanatorium soon had a "waiting list of almost one hundred persons"[26] and gradually expanded its patient population to include many with terminal disease.

Established in Pasadena in 1910, La Viña Sanatorium apparently followed a similar trajectory. The 1922 annual report noted that "advanced as well as incipient cases are admitted."[27] Although the facility had cared "for some who have not recovered their health," the report emphasized a follow-up study demonstrating "that many are living useful lives."[28]

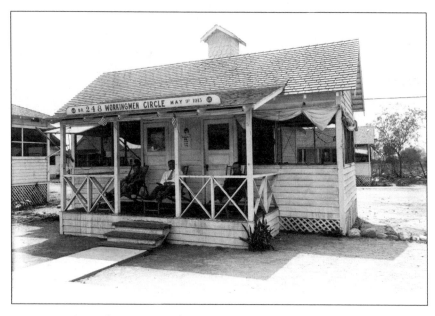

Figure 6.   An early cottage at the Sanatorium of the Jewish Consumptive Relief Association

Courtesy of the Archive of the City of Hope.

The foundational story of the Sanatorium of the Jewish Consumptive Relief Association (later the City of Hope) takes somewhat different forms, but all versions agree that the death of a young tubercular garment worker on a downtown sidewalk so aroused the compassion of members of the Jewish community that they vowed to establish a place where even the most destitute consumptive could find good care.[29] We have seen, however, that plans to establish a free sanatorium had provoked vehement hostility from wealthy Jews. And even the most ardent supporters emphasized the need to safeguard the broader community, not only tend the sick. Dr. Leon Shulman wrote that the goal was "to protect those free from the ravages of the white plague, to see that the unfortunate, homeless tubercular patients do not further spread the disease."[30]

The beginning of the new facility was hardly auspicious. The announcement of an impending county ordinance to restrict the establishment of unpopular institutions forced the Jewish Consumptive Relief Association to open the sanatorium before it was ready. A storm soon destroyed the two tents erected in Duarte (twenty miles east of the city), and the four patients were removed to the county hospital.[31] Nevertheless, the association persevered. Despite the opposition of more conservative Jewish philanthropies, the association launched a national appeal. As funds poured in from auxiliary groups throughout the nation, construction of permanent buildings began and the patient population grew. By 1926, the facility included thirty-one buildings and cottages housing 120 patients.[32] In 1919 the association added a convalescent facility, the Ex-Patients Home, in Belvedere. The two facilities merged in 1928, becoming the largest private tuberculosis institution in Southern California.[33]

Private sanatoriums were never expected to care for the majority of needy people. That responsibility, advocates insisted, lay with the state government. By the early twentieth century, the East Coast provided numerous examples California could follow. As the *Southern California Practitioner* wrote in February 1905, the Massachusetts state sanatorium had been in existence seven years, New York had opened Ray Brook Sanatorium the previous summer, Rhode Island's buildings were close to completion, and three other states had either selected sites or appropriated funds. "Laying aside the sentimental part of the question," a California institution would prevent most people "from ever reaching the advanced stage of the disease, wherein they become the greatest danger." Such a facility also "could be a great economic factor." "It must be remembered," the journal stressed, "that the great majority of cases of tuberculosis develop between the ages of fifteen and thirty-five, the best part of the human life, when the individual is of the most value to his family and to the state. If three-fourths of these people could be restored to their earning capacity, it would be a great saving to the municipality and to the state."[34] Three years later, however, Governor George C. Pardee vetoed a bill appropriating $200,000 for the construction of a state sanatorium.[35]

The 1910 election of Governor Hiram Warren Johnson, the Progressive Republican candidate, spurred the adoption of an array of social welfare measures. One of the first enabled the State Board of Health to appoint a commission to investigate "the tuberculosis problem of California" and "determine the best means for its eradication."[36] Prominent Los Angeles tuberculosis experts served on both the five-member executive committee and the fifty-member advisory board. Like many other Progressive-era documents, the reports relied heavily on economic rhetoric and emphasized the need to conserve labor power. Sir Ronald Ross, the head of the Liverpool (England) School of Tropical Medicine, had presented a powerful argument in favor of public funding, and he was quoted over and over. "For economic reasons alone," Ross had asserted, "governments are justified in spending, for the prevention of diseases, a sum equal to the loss which those diseases inflict on the people."[37] A crude cost/benefit analysis helped make the case for California. Tuberculosis caused approximately 5,000 deaths annually in the state, mostly among men and women in their most productive years (25–44). The average "commercial value" of their lives (estimated by subtracting their maintenance from their salaries) was $1,700. The total loss of life thus amounted to $8,500,000. Because the disease typically lasted four years, there were at least 20,000 tuberculosis patients, few of whom could work after the first year. Their loss of earnings was approximately $3,000,000. When medical costs were added to those figures, the total annual expenditures on tuberculosis came to $22,000,000.[38] County hospitals and other public facilities caring for tuberculosis patients spent just $500,000 a year. "Business policy" would suggest dramatically increasing that amount.[39]

The first practical result of the commission's work was the establishment of a Bureau of Tuberculosis in the State Board of Health in 1915. Edythe Tate-Thompson served as its director for more than two decades. A forthright, judgmental woman who often incited controversy and clashed frequently with local officials, Tate-Thompson had arrived from Wisconsin the previous year to direct the California Tuberculosis Association.[40] In addition to taking aggressive action to stem the tide of indigent invalids, she wielded substantial power over local programs. Soon after her appointment, the legislature decided not to establish a state sanatorium but rather to provide a $3-a-week subsidy to counties for every indigent patient in an approved facility. Tate-Thompson thus traveled frequently throughout the state inspecting all public hospitals and sanatoriums to ensure that they conformed to bureau requirements. Because she had authority to recommend the discontinuance of the subsidy for any institution, her opinions carried enormous weight.

Los Angeles County responded quickly to the subsidy law, beginning construction of Olive View Sanatorium in the northern part of the San Fernando Valley in 1918 and admitting ninety-five patients in 1920. The first long-term superintendent was William Henry Bucher, who held the appointment until his death in 1934.[41] Although originally created as a branch of the county hospital, Olive View became a separate entity under the Department of Charities in 1924.[42] Nevertheless, the two facilities remained closely linked. Together they preserved the distinction between the deserving and undeserving poor. Like the overwhelming majority of public sanatoriums, Olive View initially admitted only curable cases (typically considered the most worthy), leaving terminal patients in the far less desirable county hospital.[43] And Olive View always seemed to shine especially brightly when contrasted with the older institution. Located four miles from the nearest town, the sanatorium was able to segregate its clientele from the rest of the population, unlike the hospital, situated close to the downtown of a rapidly growing city. Equally important, the sanatorium provided the kind of environment believed to facilitate healing. While noise and dirt infiltrated the hospital from the surrounding industry, the sanatorium took its name from its site in foothills overlooking a large olive ranch. A 1925 report praised Olive View's "pure air and the freedom from choice and disturbance of any kind," which created "the best natural conditions humanly possible to obtain for the patients."[44] Tate-Thompson proclaimed the new facility "a paradise."[45]

Nevertheless, the location had serious disadvantages. Because street car service did not extend that far, administrators had difficulty attracting staff.[46] The unpaved road from town subjected sick patients to considerable "shaking up."[47] And, like many structures in the newly developed Los Angeles hills, the wooden dormitories were extremely vulnerable to fire.[48] In 1923 Bucher warned the Board of Supervisors, "We have had at various times brush fires close to the institution, and one or two of sufficient gravity as to threaten the buildings, but as they happened at opportune times they were controlled. Under unfavorable circumstances, such as a terrifically high wind blowing, as happens in this section, no hope of saving the buildings could be entertained, and it is doubtful if with all our efforts, more than a small number of the patients could be saved from destruction."[49] Although the board instituted some of the reforms Bucher requested, fire remained a major concern.[50]

In 1921 Tate-Thompson forwarded a letter to the Board of Trustees from a patient who wrote "to tell of the wonderful treatment we are receiving here . . . we all realize that while the Doctor is a martinet, he has the best interest of every patient at heart."[51] But Tate-Thompson also pointed out that only a greatly enlarged facility could relieve the terrible overcrowding in the county hospital, and she continually pressed the board to construct new buildings, increase the patient population, and hire additional staff.[52] The board agreed, and the following year it inaugurated a building program which "was to last," in the words of a later report, "almost without interruption until 1931."[53] As new wards opened, patient capacity grew, reaching 917 in 1931.[54] The number of nurses increased from 82 in 1925 to 231 in 1930.[55] Other developments expanded the range of services. A laboratory was established in 1926.[56] After the opening of a surgical unit in 1929, collapse therapy began to occupy a prominent place in the medical regime. (A painful procedure first devised in the 1890s, the operation typically involved the collapse of the diseased lung through either the introduction of air into the pleural cavity or the removal of the ribs; the surgery became extremely popular between 1920 and 1950.)[57] By 1935, according to the sanatorium director, more that half of the patients received "some form of collapse treatment."[58]

The emphasis on transforming patients into workers meant that education and rehabilitation programs were considered almost as important as medical treatment. The Board of Education built a school for children on the grounds and assigned a full-time occupational therapy teacher to the sanatorium for adults.[59]

As at Barlow, patients were expected to work as soon as possible. Bucher's biographer and successor, Dr. Emil Bogen, explained, "There comes a time in the sanatorium life of many a patient, during which work is the most essential part of his cure. If it is not available he runs the risk of assuming an attitude that the world owes him all he can get, anyway, and any energy he has he will expend in devising means to escape work."[60] In convalescent camps, the patient who "rather likes being coddled" was taught to "stand on his own feet."[61] Rather than receive meals and lodging "for nothing," the patients were expected to contribute two hours of work; that time was gradually increased until the staff felt "sure they can safely return to civil life."[62] For patients who could not "return to their former positions," the State Bureau of Rehabilitation established a school offering courses in such fields as bookkeeping and stenography.[63]

But even business courses were far too arduous for most Olive View residents. Bogen acknowledged, "The pressure from the large number of patients needing treatment in Los Angeles County became so great that it was necessary to abandon the original plan of taking only early cases."[64] Of the sixty-six new patients admitted in April 1928, fifty (75 percent) had "far advanced" disease.[65] Olive View reports continued to focus on the few patients who had been restored to workforce capacity. Widely publicized homecoming days featured the most successful.[66] Nevertheless, as one of the first nurses recalled, "It was really a terminal place." Many patients were "hemorrhaging and very, very ill." "They were coming because they knew that it was the end for them."[67]

Tate-Thompson's primary concern was not the level of disease of the clients but rather their place of origin, and in 1924 she urged the Board of Supervisors to restrict admission to people who had lived in the county at least a year. "Otherwise," she warned, "because, first, of the depression in the East and second, because of the migration of ex-service men and their families," Los Angeles would be "running the type of hospital that is now being run at Duarte where patients from all over the United States are cared for on the day of arrival." (Duarte was the site of the Jewish Consumptive Relief Association's facility, which, contrary to the wishes of the Jewish elite, welcomed patients from all parts of the country.) She continued by noting that there was a "tremendous demand for beds everywhere," and counties throughout California had discovered that "whenever a new hospital is opened that people are very apt to try and take advantage of it." The tuberculosis wards of the county hospital could accommodate "non-resident cases," thus offering "some protection for Olive View."[68] Her arguments apparently swayed the board, which instituted the requirement she recommended.

But Tate-Thompson remained dissatisfied. In 1929 she wrote again, now demanding two years residence in the county. Her argument was that "many people are being admitted to Olive View at the expense of the taxpayers of Los Angeles county who come to Los Angeles for their health, and many of them with the deliberate intention of going into Olive View." "You have, as you know, one of the best tuberculosis sanatoria in the world," she added, but there was "no reason . . . why it should be operated at the expense of the taxpayers of Los Angeles county for people who have . . . contributed nothing towards the support of Los Angeles, either as far as work is concerned or their owning property is concerned." Tate-Thompson did not "blame any patient or their friends for making every effort to place them at Olive View but at the same time there must be a limit to the number of beds that Los Angeles county or any other county maintains for the support of the indigent tuberculous patients in the community."[69]

This time local officials exploded in fury. Superintendent of Charities W. H. Holland reminded the board that nonresidents were admitted only to the county hospital, which was "required to perform this service for any person in need, regardless of length of residence."[70] Lucy M. Rice, Olive View placement supervisor, strongly doubted that people came to Los Angeles "with the deliberate intention" of entering that institution. Most patients "know nothing about the Sanatorium until they sought medical attention after their arrival." And Rice pointed out that stricter residence requirements would thwart efforts "to control or check the spread" of a dangerous disease. "Applicants can be denied admission to Olive View, to be sure, but that does not alter the situation as far as the patient is concerned in relation to his family or the community. He is just as much in need of medical and nursing care and just as infectious as though he had been here more than one or two years."[71] Although the depression soon would precipitate dramatic changes at Olive View, the one-year requirement remained in effect.

Out-patient services (clinics and public health nurses) were the responsibility of the two local health departments. The sparse information available suggests that, like the state government, city and county officials had to be prodded to take action and that most early programs were seriously deficient. In 1915 the *Southern California Practitioner* noted that the one "tuberculosis nurse thus far maintained by the city was . . . employed as a result of the efforts of Dr. George H. Kress," who "after a struggle of some months" convinced the City Council to allocate funds.[72] A leading tuberculosis physician, Kress had served on the executive committee of the state commission investigating tuberculosis control in 1911 and directed the Society for the Study and Prevention of Tuberculosis. Increasing the size of the nursing staff required an even greater struggle. In December 1913, the society sent a petition with more than 250 signatures representing "a large proportion of the tax-paying merchants of Los Angeles" to the City Council, urging it to hire more nurses. In typical fashion, the society invoked the example of the

East Coast and emphasized the goal of promoting public safety. The cover letter stated, "New York, with 165 tuberculosis nurses, has reduced the tuberculosis cases and deaths more than one-fourth. Following this lead, a number of eastern cities, notably Buffalo, Cleveland, Boston and Baltimore, have markedly increased their number of tuberculosis nurses. After studying the local condition, in Los Angeles, it would seem that we ought to have about the same number as Buffalo, seventeen." Because the "chief duty" of tuberculosis nurses was to educate patients "in hygiene and sanitation," they helped to reduce the "menace" consumptives posed to those with whom they come in contact."[73] When the City Council rejected the appeal, the society took the issue directly to the voters. In the 1914 municipal election, an ordinance was passed mandating the employment of one tuberculosis nurse for every one hundred reported cases of tuberculosis in the city; as a result, the number of nurses jumped to twenty.[74]

The Society for the Study and Prevention of Tuberculosis also provided financial support for the eight clinics established by the City Health Department between 1906 and 1926.[75] Most were open just a few hours a week.[76] A 1928 report noted that they lacked adequate staff and equipment.[77]

The County Department of Health gained national recognition for its large health centers established after 1927, offering both preventive and curative care. Its first health centers, however, were unimpressive operations, consisting of no more than a few rooms and offering a very limited range of services; tuberculosis clinics typically were held a couple of hours one or two days a week.[78] Like the city clinics, the first county facilities relied heavily on private funding. The department's 1920 report listed nine health centers that opened the past year. One was located in the company town established by the Simons Brick Company.[79] Three others were in the housing developments built by growers' associations in San Dimas, LaVerne, and Glendora,[80] Other organizations supporting the centers included local parent teacher association, churches, and Red Cross branches.[81] By 1923 the number of health centers had increased to twenty-four.[82] The county also employed a few nurses to visit tubercular patients at home; a 1928 report concluded, however, that the staff was "considerably smaller" than needed to render "really adequate service to . . . the citizens of the County."[83]

Defining eligibility was even more critical for out-patient services than for institutional ones. The hospital accommodated many nonresidents who were denied admission to the sanatorium, but there was no safety valve for patients excluded from clinics and nursing care. A 1927 county case involving a Mexican railroad worker crystallized the issues. One month after arriving from Kansas, the worker applied for both tuberculosis and venereal disease care at the San Fernando Health Center. Expressing her dilemma in a letter to John L. Pomeroy, the director of the County Department of Health, the health-center social worker noted that the case struck at the heart of the conflict between the need to protect public safety and the imperative to contain public spending: "If we refuse this man treatment, and he cannot afford it in private practice, he may become a public health menace. On the other hand, if we accept him we are establishing a poor precedent in a taxpayers' institution."[84] Pomeroy referred the letter to the county counsel, who wrote that although no law required counties to provide medical treatment to nonresidents, there also was "no adequate legal means whereby the county may rid itself of the presence of such indigents, or escape the necessity of furnishing medical attention in case such indigents become a public health menace." The county could agree to pay all the expenses to transport indigents to their homes but could not compel them to leave. As a result, the county was "not in a very satisfactory position to protect itself against the imposition of the nonresident indigent sick who insist upon visiting with us indefinitely and against our will."[85] The clinics continued to accept migrants with TB as soon as they arrived in the county.

Although the Los Angeles Tuberculosis Association frequently publicized its work funding out-patient services and agitating for increased government expenditures, the organization's proudest achievement was its own facility, the Preventorium of Los Angeles. The first preventorium had been established in 1909 by Alfred Hess, a New York City pediatrician, for poorly nourished children who had been exposed to infection at home. His New Jersey facility accommodated 150 children between the ages of four and fourteen, who stayed an average of three months.[86] "The plan of treatment is simple," Hess wrote, "plenty of good food, a twenty-four-hour day in the open air, an intimate acquaintanship [sic] with the fields and woods, and a practical lesson in cleanliness and hygiene."[87] By the late 1920s, there were forty-five preventoriums with a total of 2,783 beds in various parts of the United States.[88] Enthusiasm for those institutions waned during the late 1930s, and the great majority had closed by 1950.[89]

Unlike more U.S. preventoriums, the one in Los Angeles served only boys. Established as a day camp in 1916, it was converted into a year-round facility in 1925. Ninety boys ages seven through fourteen were admitted for four-month periods. The construction of the San Gabriel Dam forced the institution to move to Monrovia in 1933; it ceased operation five years later.[90]

As befitted a facility serving physically vulnerable children, the preventorium instituted lengthy rest hours, served healthy meals, and provided regular medical examinations. Nurses carefully monitored the boys throughout their stays. The preventorium also hired teachers to provide the lessons the residents missed at school.[91] In other ways, however, the facility bore a remarkable similarity to other

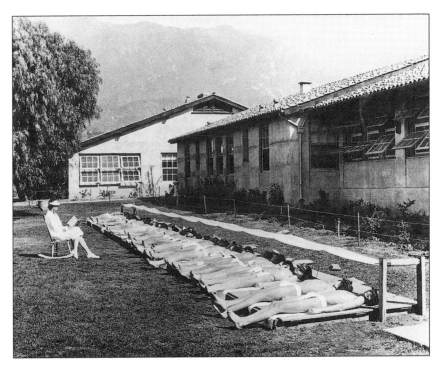

Figure 7.   Boys sunbathing at the Preventorium of Los Angeles, 1928
Courtesy of Photograph Collection, Los Angeles Public Library.

early twentieth century organizations for boys, most notably Ernest Thompson Seton's Woodcraft Indians and its successor, the Boy Scouts of America. As one historian writes, "These organizations meant to introduce coddled boys to the wilderness, to competition, to hardy play, and strenuous virtue."[92] That regime must have seemed especially critical for boys deemed at high risk of tuberculosis. Despite the dramatic changes in the understanding of the etiology of that disease since George Weeks attempted to cure himself by turning himself into a western "cowboy," reigning notions of manliness continued to inform medical advice. A recent finding had made it imperative to focus on the power of individuals to repel the disease—although the germ affected 90 percent of the population, only a small minority developed symptoms. Experts thus turned their attention to individual resistance. "More often than not," two historians note, "doctors spoke simply of a person's 'strength,' the 'toughness' of their lungs, and their 'general vitality'; indeed, the open air treatment at this time was often spoken of . . . as being designed to 'harden off' patients."[93] "Strength" and

"toughness," of course, were key components of early twentieth-century masculinity, and the Preventorium of Los Angeles worked hard to develop them in its
residents.

Although the preventorium carefully avoided the most strenuous physical
activities, moderate exercises and organized sports were essential features of the
treatment regimen. Competition was encouraged throughout the day. Even bed
making, "the most popular indoor sport," provided an occasion. As a 1927
report stated, "Rivalry is keen between the groups over the speed-and-efficiency
record."[94] "Playing Indian" was as important in the preventorium as in many contemporary boys' organizations.[95] Archery was a central activity, and boys were
encouraged to "wear an absolute minimum of clothing." "Without an exception,"
a report noted, "the semi-nude plan has resulted in benefit to the child; before
he leaves he is as brown and hardy as a little Indian."[96] Another key goal was to
weaken the ties between boys and their "over-indulgent" mothers. Among the
traits the facility sought to expunge were unassertiveness and reticence; undesirable behaviors included crying and giggling.[97]

Despite the enormous focus on establishing residence requirements to reduce
patient demand, many observers acknowledged that client response to the tuberculosis program tended to be far less enthusiastic than expected. Report after
report complained about patients who missed clinic appointments, rebuffed public health nurses, and either rejected recommendations to enroll in institutions or
departed prematurely.[98] Knowing little about the population they purported to
serve, health authorities used such actions to confirm negative stereotypes. Clients
failed to comply with public health advice because they were "ignorant,"
"vicious," and "overcome by inertia."[99] They disregarded clinic appointments to
pursue "amusements," a serious charge at a time when reformers labeled most
city pleasures "evil."[100] "Prejudice," "superstition," and "dread" retarded hospital
placement.[101]

In a study of New York City's pioneering tuberculosis control program, I
found that many patient actions that seemed irrational to middle-class observers
made sense from the client perspective.[102] Available records are much scantier
in Los Angeles, but they suggest that patients in that metropolis rejected tuberculosis services for similar reasons.

Although public health nurses and social workers prided themselves in
demonstrating unlimited "tact" and "sympathy,"[103] some acknowledged that
they "scolded" clients who failed to heed public health.[104] One noted that clients
often resented all "outside interference," no matter how kindly intended.[105] Poor
people also lacked the resources necessary to comply with medical recommendations. Nourishing food and airy apartments were expensive. Dirt was inevitable

in overcrowded and dilapidated homes.[106] And all advice implied the superiority of white, middle-class culture.

Clinic attendance entailed other problems. People with advanced disease were extremely weak. As a social work student wrote, "Even riding both ways on the street cars, the clients are tired from the trip of a few blocks, to say nothing of the exhaustion from attending the clinic."[107] And many patients lived much farther away, especially in sparsely populated areas.[108] The major city clinic was located on the tenth floor of a building, requiring patients to climb as many flights of stairs.[109] After reaching clinics, patients often had to wait hours in noisy, overcrowded, and dirty rooms.[110] Some were told to return the next day.[111]

The determination of patients to avoid the miserable conditions of the county hospital may need little explanation. But patients also had good reasons for refusing to enter higher-quality institutions. All facilities separated sick people from home, subjected them to harsh regimes (even a grateful patient, we recall, described Olive View's doctor as a "martinet"), and forced them to experience the sights and sounds of serious illness and death. A woman who entered Olive View in 1929 recalled, "One night I heard a girl drown. It was a tragic thing, her lungs just filled up and filled up . . . I knew what was happening . . . She was drowning in her own fluid. There was no hope, nothing they could do."[112] Many patients were convinced they could receive better care from family members at home.[113]

In-patient care also created problems for families. The institutionalization of breadwinners devastated households financially.[114] Women often tried to enter the labor force when their husbands became ill, but some never had worked before and hesitated to do so. After her husband quit work to enter a sanatorium, Pauline Schweitzer told the Jewish Social Service Bureau "she was ashamed of the fact that she was forced to support the family."[115] Child-care responsibilities kept other women out of the labor force. And few working women could replace their husbands' wages. When Esther Weiss's tubercular husband was "obliged to discontinue work," she found employment "as an operator in the needle trade" earning $65 a month. The family's monthly expenditure, however, totaled $95.74.[116] Home work paid much less. William F. Snow, the secretary of the California State Board of Health, reported in 1911 that "a mother may bring in 1½ to 2 per cent [of the income needed to support a family] through mending or other home piecework, and 6 to 8 per cent through taking in boarders. The minor children may collectively bring in 8 to 10 per cent more. A possible 20 per cent therefore of the minimum necessary income for a family may be supplied by a mother and her children without sacrificing her home or the schooling of the children."[117]

The departure of women deprived families of their primary caregivers. One social worker reported that although Rebecca Sklar had "been ill for several years suffering with tuberculosis," she "refused hospitalization on the basis that she could not leave her young children without care."[118] The many L.A. residents who were recent arrivals tended to lack the support networks that might have been available at home to take in children.[119] Relatives who offered assistance were not always acceptable.[120] The Jewish Social Service Society occasionally supplied housekeepers to provide child care when mothers went to the hospital or sanatoriums; more commonly, children were sent to foster homes or institutions. In 1910, Jewish philanthropists established the Orphans' Home, which accommodated the children of many women with TB.[121] But it was not easy for women to relinquish their offspring. Although administrators touted the high quality of care they offered, mothers remained suspicious.[122] Children with behavior problems were denied admission.[123] And the Orphans' Home catered only to the Jewish community; other parents had fewer options.

Moreover, although institutionalization relieved families of the burden of nursing very sick people, it also imposed new anxieties and responsibilities. Visiting patients in Olive View, for example, was exceedingly difficult. Instructions for reaching the facility stated that people should take a bus or Pacific Electric car to San Fernando and then proceed by "private conveyance."[124] Automobile ownership grew rapidly during the 1920s, reaching half of the adult population by 1925,[125] but the low-income households most likely to have members in Olive View were among the last to achieve that status. Without the freeways that would later span Los Angeles, even car owners had to spend half a day traveling to the facility from some parts of the county.

Children had no contact with their institutionalized parents. In an oral history interview, Emilia Casteñeda de Valenciana recalled her mother's illness: "One of the neighbors finally decided to take her to the hospital, so she could have a checkup. They didn't let her return home because they said that she was too sick. She had T.B. Then I never saw her anymore because children weren't allowed to go into the sanitarium to see their sick parents." Although Emilia and her brother went to the sanatorium with their father, "we couldn't see her. We had to keep our distance from the building. We used to spend our time just playing around on the property, but not too close because they didn't allow us to even go close to the porch where you could at least put your head against the screen door to peek in at your relative. We weren't even allowed to do that because they were afraid that we'd catch the disease."[126]

Communication between visits was a problem regardless of age. Mary Helen Ponce recalled that when her brother lay dying in Olive View, her parents

lived nearby and thus could see him regularly, but because they lacked a tele-
phone, they had to rely on a neighborhood grocer for news.[127] Emilia Castañeda
de Valenciana noted how she learned of her mother's death:

> My mother died on a Sunday morning. I was making my First Communion.
> That's why I thought I remembered the date. Since we didn't have a phone,
> we had given a neighbor's phone number to the sanitarium. Who could
> afford to have a phone in those days? Just the people who had money or
> who had employment. Not us. Anyway, the sanitarium had tried to call
> the neighbor, but she was gone somewhere for the day, and she didn't get
> home until late in the afternoon. My mother had died in the morning . . . I
> didn't find out until after mass that my mother had died . . . I remember one
> of the girls in the neighborhood first told me that my mother had died,
> which was a shock, especially on such a happy occasion. When something
> like this happens happiness turns to sadness.[128]

And then there was the lien, the agreement property owners were required to
sign promising to reimburse the county for the cost of care in either of its facilities.
Because patients with TB typically remained in institutions for extended periods,
the costs ($2.25 a day and $67.50 a month) quickly mounted. The lien could be
applied to future home ownership and thus affected the many renters who hoped
to accumulate enough capital to purchase their dwellings.[129] In some cases,
county officials confiscated family homes long after patients had died.[130]

The lien was an especially cruel requirement in a metropolis which had long
advertised the ability to purchase a house as a major attraction. Although we tend
to associate home ownership with the most privileged social groups, rates also
were unusually high among African Americans, Mexicans, and low-income
whites.[131] Carmen Armendarez noted that her mother "needed to raise $40 for
the down payment" for a home near Claremont. "She used every cent she had
saved from the walnut crop to buy her dream house." The dwelling was "small
and *very* modest," but the mother was "thrilled" because "she finally had a place
[where] her children [could run] about freely without the restrictions imposed by
their landlords in their previous homes."[132]

Long-term institutionalization could abort such dreams. Fernando
Valenzuela lost his home to pay a $2,100 medical bill for one of his children; as a
result, he and his five sons departed to work in a Fresno pickle factory, leaving the
mother and two daughters in Los Angeles. His ultimate goal was to earn enough
to purchase another house.[133] Not everyone agreed to sign the lien. According to
a letter from Superintendent of Charities W. H. Holland to the Board of
Supervisors, a "day laborer" who owned a "little five-room frame house in

Belvedere valued at $1,250" refused "to allow the county to place a lien on his property toward his son's care at Olive View."[134] In another case, Holland asked permission to waive the property restrictions for a man who had "lost everything he had except the equity in his property as a result of continued sickness." Visiting the home, Holland "found the family absolutely destitute." The "interest and the taxes were due" and the family had "nothing upon which to live." If the board allowed the family to retain the property after the man entered Olive View, they could find a renter and "live on the income and gradually pay off current indebtedness."[135] Rather than appealing to county officials, most home owners in desperate straits must simply have rejected offers of admission to county facilities. Antonia Monatones recalled going with her father to sign a lien on the property before her brother could enter Olive View. Fearing that his stay would exhaust the family's savings and thus result in the loss of the home, her brother left early. After he died, the family sold the house for $2,500; the county took $500.[136]

In short, the tuberculosis program often met opposition because it imposed serious hardships even while promising protection from a terrible scourge. But if we can explain patient resistance, we should be wary of overstating it. Most reports come from officials, doctors, nurses, and social workers who had an interest in exaggerating the extent to which patients failed to adhere to the recommended regime. Attributing poor outcomes to noncompliance reinforced negative attitudes about poor people with tuberculosis and diverted attention from the ineffectiveness of available therapies.

Moreover, long waiting lists for institutional beds and overcrowded clinics remind us that the tuberculosis program garnered enormous support, even while generating hostility. Indeed, as the population exploded during the boom of the twenties and access problems accelerated, health officials increasingly blamed low-income patients for overutilizing expansive services rather than rejecting them. Officials who added the cost of monetary relief to that of medical care were especially likely to complain that families with tuberculosis drained government coffers.

Two East Coast studies sought to explain why tuberculosis patients represented a high proportion of the recipients of financial assistance. A 1913 report of New York families on relief at TB clinics discussed twenty-one families in which the man was living but suffering from the disease. Only four of those men continued to hold their jobs, seven were unemployed, and ten had irregular jobs with lower pay.[137] The same year, a Boston study of 256 living men who had visited a tuberculosis dispensary during the preceding five years found that they had lost an average of 89.3 weeks of work (more than one-third of their work time).[138]

Recent scholarship in disability studies can help us understand why tuberculosis led so frequently to withdrawal from the labor force. A key tenet of that field is that the problems encountered by disabled people stem as much from social arrangements (including prejudice and the structure of work) as from individual impairments.[139] As information about the communicable nature of tuberculosis spread, employers fired workers suspected of harboring the disease. Even former patients could be dismissed once their histories were revealed.[140] Upperclass people refrained from bringing washing or sewing to women in affected families; boarders fled homes with the disease.

In addition, tubercular patients often could find only jobs that imposed excessive physical burdens. When advancing disease prevented booster-journalist Charles Willard from fulfilling the demands of his position as secretary of the Municipal League, his friends crafted an editorial position he could do at home, and occasionally even from bed.[141] Manual workers were not so lucky. In 1911, Barlow Sanatorium's resident physician wrote, "When our patients reach that point in their recovery at which it would be possible for them to do some light work and thereby support themselves, we are not able to advise them to leave the Sanatorium, for the reason that it is impossible for them to find work which is within the limits of safety."[142] An official of the Los Angeles County Department of Charities complained in 1923 that tuberculosis patients "are referred to us by the clinics as being able to do light work and we don't know what that light work is. We haven't got it for them to do."[143]

The less strenuous jobs that existed rarely paid a living wage. After receiving a tuberculosis diagnosis in 1925, Daniel Smith, a Tennessee carpenter, moved to Los Angeles. When his condition worsened and he no longer could work at his usual occupation, he found employment as a night watchman. That job allowed him to rest during his shift, but he did not earn enough to support his family.[144] The executive secretary of the Los Angeles Tuberculosis Association discussed the case of a "discouraged" woman whose "tuberculosis condition was quiescent and wanted employment which would enable her to make a modest living which would not break her health again." She had "been forced to work far beyond her strength in laundries and in janitor service after which experiences she would not be able to be out of bed for several days." The association "arranged for her to do a few hours each day in a nursing home." Her wages, however, were scanty.[145]

Tuberculosis could propel family members as well as patients out of the workforce. One woman applied for assistance when she relinquished her job as a domestic servant to nurse her tubercular husband at home.[146] Another needed help because she remained unemployed to care for both her elderly father and her sister "suffering with tuberculosis."[147]

In one way, families visited by the disease were fortunate. Financial assistance programs historically have singled out poor people who were sick or disabled as especially deserving.[148] Because virtually all applicants claimed impairments that prevented them from working, it was important to present a precise and verifiable diagnosis. A tuberculosis label fit that description.[149]

One historian points out, however, that the high premium placed on self-reliance meant that policies which excused the "'deserving' disabled poor" from work simultaneously "stigmatized and marginalized" them.[150] All applicants for assistance had to undergo humiliating investigations, including home visits and interviews with employers, relatives, and neighbors.

Furthermore, little aid was available for anyone in early twentieth-century Los Angeles. Unlike most American cities, the metropolis lacked a major philanthropic organization. After the Associated Charities (formed in 1893) disbanded in 1914, the only private relief agencies were the Jewish Social Service Bureau and Catholic Charities, both of which restricted eligibility to their own communities.[151] The director of Medical Social Work in the County Department of Health later recalled, "The theory was that you went to the agency to apply for aid according to your religion. If you didn't happen to belong to any particular religious organization and the county refused you perhaps you did not get aid."[152]

It was all too easy to be rejected by the county. Its general relief program, administered by the Department of Charities, was extremely parsimonious.[153] A 1915 investigation reported that the department's policy was "to assist only when no other resource is left, that is, in cases of absolute destitution, and to give only sufficient aid to barely provide food and shelter."[154] As observers frequently noted, tuberculosis was a major cause of dependence. By the late 1920s, the county aided 1,338 people "because of tuberculosis in the family or because of the death of the breadwinner from tuberculosis."[155] Together those groups represented 17 percent of the county's clients.[156] Patients with TB received special assistance, including additional stipends for milk and eggs, new beds, and occasionally even rent for larger and airier apartments. Case workers sent by the department visited patients at home, partially compensating for the dearth of public health nurses. Those visits, however, were few and far between, and even with the additional food, most families remained at starvation levels.[157]

One other option for families with tuberculosis was to apply for state aid. Although the mothers' pension law passed in 1913 restricted eligibility to widows, a 1921 amendment extended the law to women whose husbands were unable to work. Each minor child received a stipend of $10 a month, another essential benefit, though one too small to lift most families out of poverty.

Anxious to deflect attention from the shortcomings of their own programs, health officials often blamed high TB rates on the stinginess of welfare services. In a 1930 report, Edythe Tate-Thompson wrote that "for years" the Bureau of Tuberculosis "has kept at relief agencies to increase the family budget where tuberculosis is a problem. It is nothing short of the stupidest, most wasteful economy to spend the money to restore a patient's health in a sanatorium and then on his return either decrease the family budget or refuse to add an extra amount of aid for the patient. We could increase our turnover in the sanatoria very much faster if we could be sure this could and would be done."[158] But amounts that seemed miserly to Tate-Thompson and clients appeared exorbitant to many tax-payers. Ironically, Tate-Thompson helped to inflame public opinion by publishing reports highlighting the economic burdens tuberculosis patients imposed as recipients of monetary assistance as well as health-care services. Her comments became especially strident as Mexicans and other "outsiders" began to represent an ever-increasing proportion of the beneficiaries.

Chapter 4

"Outsiders"

White Americans at the turn of the twentieth century took as a matter of faith that physical strength and vigor underlay their social and political supremacy. Photographs of muscular, healthy soldiers justified the nation's first foray into imperialism.[1] Feminist writer Charlotte Perkins Gilman sought to advance women's position by declaring that "the dominant soul—the clear strong accurate brain, the perfect service of a health body" belonged not just to one gender but to the entire race.[2] The heavy-weight boxing victory of African American Jack Johnson over white Jim Jeffries shocked primarily by upsetting cherished notions about racial superiority.[3]

Similar ideas infused the Los Angeles promotional campaign. According to the boosters, whites already had won the Darwinian race for survival. Since losing the protection of the missions, California Indians had begun to die out.[4] Because the Chinese lacked immunity to consumption, they quickly succumbed to the disease.[5] Above all, the contrast between Anglo-Saxon energy and Mexican lassitude demonstrated the fit between whites and the land. In 1880, Los Angeles was still a "sleepy semi-Mexican *pueblo* of 11,000." Its homes were "mostly of *adobe*, or sun-dried brick." Its streets were "unpaved and few even graded." Its commerce was "confined to wool and hides."[6] Within ten years, whites had increased the population fivefold, built fine roads, schools, churches, homes, and hotels, and "transformed great ranches of dry pasture land . . . into ten, twenty and forty-acre tracts of irrigated land, dotted all over with orange and lemon groves, vineyards, and deciduous orchards."[7] And, just as some crops were ideally suited to the soil and climate, so Anglo-Saxons were most likely to flourish in Southern California. While realizing the potential of the land, they themselves would grow to perfection.

Descriptions of Los Angeles as an exclusively white society helped to market its agricultural products and real estate. Even while inviting consumptives to find work in the newly planted citrus groves, the booster journal *Land of Sunshine* advertised Southern California crops this way: "Foreign oranges are grown in countries always more or less infected with cholera and other diseases, and picked and packed by dirty lazzaroni to be stowed in the unclean hold of some Italian sailing vessel, while the Southern California fruit is grown, handled and carried by clean and healthy Americans."[8] Prospective settlers were assured that they would associate only with whites. An editorial entitled "The Right Kind of People" proclaimed, "We are not compelled, as in most eastern cities, to set aside 20 to 30 per cent as speaking little or no English and caring nothing for American institutions. . . . Only the best class of immigration thus far has been attracted to this section, and the situation is likely to continue the same in the future."[9]

The desire for cheap labor shattered the dream of racial homogeneity. During the early twentieth century, the center of the growing Japanese population shifted from northern to southern California. By 1920, nearly 20,000 Japanese lived in Los Angeles County.[10] The overwhelming majority were young, single men, many of whom worked in agriculture and domestic service. Some quickly prospered, buying farms or establishing small businesses.[11] Perhaps as a result, Japanese workers occasionally received praise as well as contempt. The *Sacramento Bee* lauded them as "clearly, [sic] amiable, and industrious, having many virtues and few vices."[12] Although Charles Dwight Willard referred to the "filthy personal habits" of other "foreigners,"[13] he described a new family servant thus: "We have a jewel of a cook named Oura— a Jap—he makes everything taste so good and May says he is the most exquisitely neat and orderly person she ever knew in her life. His kitchen is like a dream of a kitchen. As a rule the Japanese are sanitary, you know."[14]

Nevertheless, the Japanese soon became the focus of a campaign of exclusion. The Asiatic Exclusion League, organized in San Francisco in 1905, inspired the San Francisco Board of Education to segregate all Asian students. Although the board rescinded that order at Theodore Roosevelt's behest, discrimination continued. In the 1907 Gentleman's Agreement, the Japanese government promised to restrict the number of laborers migrating to the United States, and in 1914 the California legislature forbade aliens from owning land.[15]

Throughout the United States, early twentieth century public health officials helped to inflame prejudice against immigrants by associating them with disease.[16] John L. Pomeroy, the director of the newly established Los Angeles County Department of Health, was no different. Despite the many laudatory comments about the cleanliness of the Japanese he must have heard, he charged them with contaminating the food supply. In 1919, he explained why he needed to hire additional food inspectors: "About 85% of the vegetables are raised by Japanese, and our evidence shows that many of these places are very unsanitary. It is vitally necessary that more officers be employed to enforce the law—if our people are to be protected against impure food and disease."[17] The phrase "our people" clearly demarcated the limits of Pomeroy's responsibility.

Two years later he wrote that, "with one exception," he could not determine the cause of typhoid fever cases. "The one exception developed at a Japanese picnic near Redondo on the 4th of July. Following this picnic cases occurred in various sections, especially around the Gardena and Lomita districts. There evidently was a typhoid carrier who helped prepare the food consumed at the picnic. As these cases occurred in Japanese who are vegetable raisers and at a time when many of the vegetables placed on the market are in a raw form, it was necessary to exercise considerable vigilance over the quarantine measures before raising, as otherwise it would have been a distinct menace to the whole county."[18] Contemporary public health literature would have alerted Pomeroy to the dangers posed by healthy carriers. In addition, because he previously had served in the New York City Department of Health, he probably followed the case of Mary Mallon (commonly known as Typhoid Mary), which preoccupied that department after her 1907 apprehension. An Irish-born cook accused of transmitting the tubercle bacilli to several families, Mallon was quarantined for twenty-five years in an isolation hospital on North Brother Island in the East River. Health officials routinely referred to her as an "Irish woman," and her ethnicity (along with her gender and social class) figured prominently in arguments for her incarceration.[19] But what is most striking about Pomeroy's account is its failure to mention the fate of the sick. Who cared for them? Were they hospitalized? Did they recover? (The disease had a case fatality rate of approximately 10 percent.)[20] His focus on white health rendered such questions irrelevant.

Pomeroy's report for 1921 stressed yet another way Japanese food handlers endangered public health: "The department feels proud of the matter relative to the protection of the people from arsenic poisoning in relation to the Japanese celery growers, since this department brought this problem to a solution before it became generally dangerous to the public. It seems that the Japanese celery growers were extremely careless in the use of excessive amounts of arsenate of lead and tri-oxide on the plants for the purpose of control of insects."[21] Although Pomeroy singled out Japanese celery growers, they were not alone. The demand

to produce the large, unblemished, brightly colored fruits and vegetables featured in agricultural fairs and advertisements encouraged most growers to add
large amounts of lead arsenate to their pesticides in 1912. The people most at risk
were the workers (many of them Japanese).[22]

The Japanese did not remain central to Pomeroy for long. As "the Mexican
problem" increasingly consumed his attention, Japanese food handlers vanished
from his reports. Building on the work of turn-of-the-century housing reformers, he linked Mexicans with various communicable diseases, and especially
with tuberculosis.

Of course, because Southern California originally was part of Mexico,
Mexicans were outsiders only in the Anglo-Saxon imagination. Available data
suggest that they represented 80 percent of the total population during the
1850s.[23] The racial composition of the region changed dramatically during the
eighties, when stories of cheap, fertile land and the balmy, healthy climate
lured white settlers from the East and Midwest. By the end of the "boom,"
whites outnumbered Mexicans four to one.[24] After the turn of the century, however, migrants slowly began to swell the size of the Mexican population. Some
were recruited by the railroads; others came to find agricultural jobs.[25] The
greatest influx occurred during the 1920s; by the end of the decade, Los Angeles
contained more Mexicans than any other U.S. city.[26]

They received none of the grudging respect accorded the Japanese. Southern
California whites routinely made what one historian calls "ugly, unreflexive
comments" about Mexicans.[27] Within a month of arriving in San Bernardino in
1886 (all of which had been spent in bed), Charles Dwight Willard felt competent to describe Mexican children as "filthy and only half-clad" and their parents as even "worse."[28] Other whites blamed Mexicans for spreading disease. In
1897, a father in Ivanhoe complained to the Board of Education, "At three separate times during the past four years my children have contracted scarlet fever,
measles, and at present one is sick with diphtheria, all of which have been the
result of defiance of sanitary regulations by the parents of children attending the
district school. This district, as you are doubtless aware, has a large Mexican population. They are grossly ignorant and reckless of all sanitary precautions necessary in contagious diseases." The father urged the board to instruct the county
health officer to "frame regulations for use in school districts and to have the
same printed in English, Spanish and any and every language necessary to bring
them within the knowledge of the people."[29]

Early twentieth-century housing reformers both drew on and reinforced
those attitudes. The primary focus of concern was the house courts inhabited
largely by Mexican workers and their families. House courts were vacant lots

owned by the railroads on which tenants constructed small shacks, typically of tin, gunny sacks, and boxes; residents shared toilets and carried water from outdoor faucets.[30] Reformers described the residents with a mixture of pity, contempt, and fear. Because the primary goal of the progressive movement in Los Angeles was to reduce the power of the Southern Pacific, it is unsurprising that reformers castigated the railway for paying low wages and charging exorbitant rents.[31] But the misfortunes of the Mexicans also were believed to derive from personal failings. Because they were "people from rural areas," they did not understand "the necessity for sanitation."[32] The shared toilets were used "indiscriminately by both sexes."[33] And the docility that made Mexicans ideal workers from the employers' point of view prevented them from protesting their lot; they seemed "contented enough living in these filthy surroundings."[34]

Because reformers' language frequently elided miserable housing and their wretched inhabitants, the line between external and personal causes of tenants' problems could never be clearly drawn.[35] When reformers stressed "the filthy walls and floors" and the "odors that assail" the visitor, they implied that Mexican tenants were dirty and smelly.[36] Moreover, dismal housing was believed to degrade the residents. After surveying the house courts' lack of sanitation, overcrowding, and flimsy construction, Dr. Titian Coffey asked in 1906, "Is it any wonder that vice, drunkenness and crime are bred under such conditions?"[37] Sickness was an equally serious problem. "Contagious and infectious diseases, diphtheria, tuberculosis and smallpox" not only afflicted the residents but were "liable to spread to an epidemic at any time."[38] Like vagrants, Mexicans appeared pathetic as well as dangerous. "There is absolutely no more pitiable picture," Coffey wrote, "than when sickness attacks such homes. . . . Here they lie, suffer and pass to the world beyond; too poor to pay for medical attention; too poor at times to pay for medicine that may be prescribed, surrounded by squalor, misery, bad air, insufficient food, and all the woes of poverty."[39] Fatalistic, ignorant, suspicious, and poverty-stricken, Mexicans quickly succumbed to the many diseases that struck them. Similar themes soon appeared in Pomeroy's accounts.

Although he confronted the overwhelming task of building a public health infrastructure for a burgeoning population spread over a vast area, his reports focused largely on the various infectious diseases associated with Mexicans. In 1916 he explained why he needed to hire public health nurses by submitting the report of a temporary nurse who had worked in Irwindale, a "Mexican village of about 63 houses" between Covina and Azusa in the San Gabriel Valley. According to the nurse, "the secretive nature of the Mexican" made it difficult to obtain "accurate records"; nevertheless, it was clear that various infectious diseases were prevalent. The one case of syphilis demonstrated that "in the crowded condition of the homes, privacy is an impossibility, and the moral tone is low indeed." The "illicit sale of liquor" occurred constantly, tending "to demoralize these people even more than poverty and natural shiftlessness." "Proper supervision" of contagious diseases was especially important because "people refuse to go to a hospital for treatment."[40]

In his letter to the Los Angeles County Board of Supervisors, Pomeroy stressed that public health nurses were needed to "protect the general public from the spread of disease" and "prevent neglect and carelessness in sanitation and hygiene"; their work therefore should not be regarded "in the nature of a charity."[41] To some extent, this comment simply reflected the scope of Pomeroy's charge. He was responsible for safeguarding population health, leaving the care of indigents to the Department of Charities. But Pomeroy also implied that, like the Japanese, the Mexicans were outside the body politic and that their health was significant only insofar as it threatened that of whites.

In 1917, Pomeroy devoted the bulk of his report to attempts to extirpate typhus fever, which struck four Mexicans in a labor camp operated by the Southern Pacific Railroad in Harold, near Palmdale. An infectious disease spread by lice, typhus was known to be prevalent in Mexico.[42] Pomeroy noted that the railroad camp was "insanitary and overcrowded and proper facilities for bathing and general hygiene don't exist." Nevertheless, he considered Mexican workers to be masters of their own fates. "The Mexican was naturally uncleanly," his "habits tended to overcrowding," and "his ignorance and prejudice, coupled with a tendency to the life of a nomad, indeed created serious obstacles in the establishment of complete control."[43] Pomeroy predicted that more cases would develop not only because of the "unsettled conditions in Mexico" but also because many Mexicans entered the United States without undergoing medical examinations. In 1891, the U.S. Public Health Service began subjecting immigrants to such examinations, excluding anyone who displayed symptoms of "loathsome and dangerous diseases." Since 1916, inspections at El Paso (the major port of entry for Mexicans into the Southwest) had been unusually rigorous; in order to eliminate typhus, officials required all Mexican immigrants to be "deloused" in a bath containing gasoline, kerosene, and vinegar.[44] Nevertheless, Pomeroy contended that the fundamental problem persisted: "Persons may slip through the border and get into the country without passing through the usual government quarantine stations." Until the federal government tightened control along the entire border with Mexico, Pomeroy would be compelled "to maintain strict regulations over the Mexican settlements throughout the county."[45]

Perhaps no event so clearly demonstrated the readiness of local officials to blame Mexicans for disease as the great flu epidemic of 1918–19, which killed more than 21 million people worldwide, the victims coming from all social strata.[46] The first reported cases in Los Angeles were aboard a ship from San Francisco.[47] Pomeroy, however, directed his response to the usual suspects. In December 1918 he wrote that he had sent two guards, one to a neighborhood near Duarte and the other to Berrytown, "where conditions among the Mexicans made it necessary to safeguard the rest of the population."[48]

Then, in October 1924, plague visited Los Angeles, killing more than thirty people, 90 percent of whom were Mexican.[49] Plague is a highly virulent disease spread by infected fleas on rats. Because the epidemic struck close to downtown, fears soon arose that whites might be affected and that bad publicity would undermine the tourist industry. Both city and state officials joined the campaign to eradicate the disease. They acted swiftly, establishing a quarantine over the affected areas, removing victims to the county hospital, disinfecting property, destroying buildings, and killing rodents.[50] As in the 1900 plague outbreak in San Francisco, prejudice as well as reigning medical beliefs informed public health practice.[51] All reports highlighted the ethnicity of the patients and the "uncleanliness" of their neighborhoods.[52]

Far more than any other disease, tuberculosis helped health officials portray Mexicans as an overwhelming problem. One reason was that TB was an endemic condition and thus the focus of sustained rather than sporadic attention; virtually every report mentioned the prevalence of the disease among Mexicans. Moreover, although victims of typhus fever, flu, and plague either died quickly or completely recovered, tuberculosis sufferers typically remained sick for years; the long-term use of expensive tuberculosis services by Mexicans helped health officials challenge the growers' contention that the population represented a cheap form of labor. And the eugenic arguments commonly employed to explain the high TB rate among Mexicans seemed to suggest that their bodies were innately inferior to those of whites.

Dr. Gladys Patric was the first to highlight the incidence of the disease in Mexican communities, reporting in 1918 that more than a third of the houses in the North Main district had at least one case.[53] The following year Pomeroy wrote, "Our local Mexicans are contributing a much larger percentage [of deaths] due to tuberculosis than their population would entitle them to."[54] The term "entitle" may simply have been Pomeroy's awkward way of stating that Mexicans were especially likely to die prematurely as a result of that disease. But the word also may have been chosen to suggest that Mexicans were outsiders who had no claim on government resources and yet made excessive demands.

To some extent health officials explained purportedly high rates of tuberculosis by pointing to the same mix of personal characteristics and external conditions implicated in the genesis of other communicable diseases. In 1923 Pomeroy explained the need for more funding for tuberculosis control by noting, "We are having an influx of Mexicans whose ideas on sanitation and housing are very different from ours."[55] An influential state report wrote, "The families of Mexicans are larger than the average American family, therefore, the danger of tuberculosis is greater because of the contacts, and the possibilities of a cure are less because of the lowered resistance of the Mexican and the factors which he has to combat, that is, living in congested districts with unavoidable over-crowding, seasonal labor, a badly balanced diet."[56]

The phrase "lowered resistance" probably referred to the widespread belief that Mexicans had unusual susceptibility to tuberculosis.[57] Although Koch's discovery had punctured the belief that consumption could be directly inherited, many experts accepted the conclusion of the British eugenicist Karl Pearson that people inherited a predisposition to the disease.[58] A related argument was that African Americans and American Indians experienced extremely high rates of tuberculosis because they were primitive people who lacked prior exposure to the disease and thus never had developed immunity.[59] Experts seeking to understand the prevalence of tuberculosis among Mexican immigrants empha-sized their Indian makeup. In a discussion of tuberculosis in the Southwest, Dr. Ernest A. Sweet, a former employee of the U.S. Public Health Service, wrote: "The Mexicans are possessed of an extremely low racial immunity, which is probably due to the large admixture of Indian blood. Their resistance has never been developed, because they have never fought the infection through succes-sive generations. Just as in children the susceptibility decreases as age increases, so in races the further removed they are from civilization, the more susceptible they are to the disease."[60] Sweet also argued that tuberculosis advanced espe-cially rapidly among Mexicans: "Recoveries are exceedingly rare, most physi-cians confessing never to have seen one, and the course is almost invariably progressively downward. A person will be about his work apparently well, suf-fer from a hemorrhage, and in four months he will be dead." By contrast, Sweet concluded, Mexicans who were "less contaminated by Indian blood" exhibited "far more resistance to the disease."[61]

The argument that Mexican bodies were especially prone to tuberculosis and succumbed rapidly to its ravages served various purposes. It linked Mexican immigrants with the Indian rather than the European population. It contributed to the growing campaign to construct Mexicans as a racial group, not simply a national one.[62] It suggested that, if Mexicans were permitted to settle in the United States, they would affect the nation's future by producing new genera-tions of "defective" individuals. And in an era that idealized strength and vigor, it enabled whites to cast Mexicans as inherently weak. More than any other group, Mexicans lived the "strenuous life" Theodore Roosevelt had advocated in his famous 1899 speech. "Ostensibly, 'The Strenuous Life' preached the virtues of military preparedness and imperialism, but contemporaries understood it as a speech about manhood," historian Gail Bederman writes. The "underlying" message was that "American manhood—both the manly race and individual white men—must retain the strength of their Indian-fighter-ancestors, or another race would prove itself more manly and overtake America in the Darwinian struggle to be the world's most dominant race."[63] Mexicans who dug hard dirt, pushed heavy wheelbarrows, climbed steep ladders to pick oranges, stood for hours under the hot sun, and rode the rails for hundreds of miles clearly exemplified vigorous masculinity. Statements about their special vulnerability to the most fearsome disease of the time helped to counter that image.

One topic conspicuously absent from discussions about the causes of high tuberculosis rates among Mexicans was the impact of harsh working conditions. Grueling physical labor for long hours most days a week could undermine resistance and thus contribute to the onset of disease. But tuberculosis traditionally has been viewed as a "house disease."[64] Experts repeatedly stressed the risk of living in overcrowded, dark, and unsanitary conditions with sick family members. Even advocates who argued that control required broad social and economic change thus tended to emphasize tenement reform rather than reducing dangers or limiting working hours.[65] Moreover, a discussion of the impact of work on Mexican bodies would have opened the discussion to a range of occupational hazards, such as high, unsteady ladders, toxic chemicals, and the killing pace, many of which posed no danger to the white population and were thus outside the purview of early twentieth-century public health. And any attempt to intrude on the workplace would have enraged employers and thus threatened whatever support they gave the fledgling health department.

Although the segregation of Mexicans was illegal in California until 1935, some occurred in Los Angeles public schools on a de facto basis.[66] Recently discovered records indicate that health officials also separated whites and Mexicans. Geography partly dictated that policy. If disease struck Mexicans in disproportionate numbers, it made sense to situate services close to their communities. Pomeroy located four of his first nine health centers in company towns established for Mexican workers in Montebello, San Dimas, Glendora, and LaVerne.[67] In 1925, he informed the Board of Supervisors of his intention to open the Maravilla Park Health Center "in the heart of the Mexican district" of Belvedere.[68] Two years later, he requested funds to establish a small clinic near Whittier "in Jimtown, a Mexican settlement of several hundred families."[69]

But Pomeroy also segregated Mexicans when they attended the same facility as whites. His 1923 report listed two child hygiene clinics at the San Fernando Health Center, one "American" and the other "Mexican."[70] The following year Pomeroy requested permission to lease space in El Monte for a new clinic, explaining: "We have no place in this town for caring for white people. One of the churches has been providing several rooms for the Mexicans. We cannot mix the races."[71]

Like school officials, Pomeroy rationalized segregation by pointing to Mexican needs and white demands. The Maravilla Park Health Center, he noted, offered programs specifically geared toward Mexicans: "There are 10,000 Mexicans in Maravilla Park and many are in need of health education."[72] He stressed that "this, of course, protects the white people very definitely."[73] Pomeroy also argued that Maravilla Park mothers could not walk as far as the Belvedere Health Center with their children.[74]

Just as segregation in education was in part a response to white fears of contamination,[75] so Pomeroy justified the opening of the center in Maravilla Park by calling attention to "public demand for the separate treatment of certain diseases which are infectious and prevalent among these people."[76] He noted in particular the "present situation with regard to plague among Mexicans."[77]

In health care, as in education, segregation meant that Mexicans received inferior accommodations. Pomeroy assured the Board of Supervisors that the Maravilla Park Health Center "will be a very inexpensive affair."[78] He originally leased a small, wooden cottage for its use. In 1928, when the Belvedere Health Center acquired a major new building, Pomeroy moved its old one to Maravilla Park, where it served as the site of that areas's health center.[79] Two years later, Pomeroy did ask for additional funds for that facility, now noting that although Maravilla Park "is a breeding place of disease," its health center had only three treatment clinics and was "housed in a small wooden, almost ramshackle, structure."

Voluntary groups also practiced discrimination. Because it was widely believed that Mexicans were especially vulnerable to tuberculosis, we might have expected the Los Angeles Tuberculosis Association to encourage Mexican boys to enter the preventorium. The notes of a member of the association's executive board, however, lists the names and nationalities of the boys enrolled in September 1928. By that date Mexicans represented half of the patients attending county clinics.[80] But of the eighty-six preventorium residents, only three (3.5 percent) were identified as Mexican.[81] Although one possibility is that Mexican parents rejected offers of preventorium stays, it is equally likely that the need to raise private funds dictated the client composition. The association's publicity played on the assumption that whites were especially deserving of help. Photographs featured white boys engaged in the facility's various health-promoting activities. One caption read: "Aren't They Worth Saving?"[82] The unstated premise was that Mexicans were not.

White observers often invoked racial stereotypes to explain Mexican resistance to whatever tuberculosis care was available. A University of Southern California social work student quoted with approval an expert who declared that "the Mexican" resembled "the Negro," a "happy-go-lucky person who is not as profoundly disturbed by the early stages of tuberculous infection as the average white."[83] Dr. Benjamin Goldberg, a staff physician in the Municipal Tuberculosis Sanatorium of Chicago and a member of the Department of Pathology and Bacteriology of the University of Illinois College of Medicine, wrote that "the Mexican is difficult to reach with public health measures. He shuns doctors and clinics and spreads infection freely in the community, until forced, by absolute physical disability, to seek help."[84] Yet another observer, identified only as a "deaconess," wrote to the Los Angeles County Board of Supervisors: "The more ignorant Mexicans all have a deep seated fear of the County Hospital—amounting to absolute horror. Many whom they have known have died there, for what are to us obvious reasons, but there is a widespread and ineradicable conviction among these people that a convenient 'black bottle' is the cause, and to save those they love from this terror, they will hide them away to die, spreading infection while they linger."[85]

To a large extent, we can understand the response of Mexicans to tuberculosis the same way we can that of other poor people—life circumstances often intruded on the ability to take remedial action. The oral history of Emilia Castañeda de Valenciana provides one example. When asked about the beginning of her mother's tuberculosis, Emilia replied, "She caught a cold, and she probably thought that she had recovered. Instead, she got worse. . . . But she couldn't stay home because she had to go to work. My dad . . . had no employment. . . . He told her to stay home, but she wouldn't listen, she had to go to work."[86]

But one factor probably made TB services especially repellent to many Mexicans. In California, as in the East, officials insisted that the adoption of "American" practices and norms was essential to the fight against disease. Thus, public health nurses visiting Mexican homes preached the importance of substituting meat and bread for rice and beans. Institutions often had formal ties to the home teacher program, a key feature of the state's Americanization campaign. A 1915 act permitted school districts to hire special teachers "to work in the homes of the pupils, instructing children and adults in matters relating to school attendance . . . in sanitation, in the English language, in household duties . . . and in the fundamental principles of the American system of government and the rights and duties of citizenship."[87] Americanization teachers also were dispatched to tuberculosis facilities. In 1922, the Los Angeles City Board of Education assigned one to work among "the foreign tuberculous patients in the County Hospital" and another to provide instruction at Olive View."[88] Patients in those institutions who were grieving the loss of their families may have deeply resented the effort to strip them of the ethnic identities that represented continuity with the past.

In addition, language barriers often impeded interaction with doctors and nurses. Extant records suggest that Pomeroy was the only official who worked hard to facilitate communication. When he justified segregated clinics by pointing to special services he provided Mexican patients, he probably was referring to the employment of Spanish-speaking nurses;[89] when none was available, he provided interpreters.[90] Perhaps as a consequence, Pomeroy ran afoul of the Americanization campaign, which viewed the ability to speak English as the prerequisite to assimilation.[91] His 1920 report explained what happened after he hired "Mrs. Amy Chavez, a Mexican girl," as an interpreter in a clinic for Mexicans in Pomona and LaVerne:

> All of a sudden there seemed to be a dropping off of the attendance. Upon investigation this was found to be caused primarily by the lack of cooperation of Mrs. Wilson, the Americanization teacher in the public schools. Trivial things were done by this Americanization department to embarrass us in many ways. One instance in particular was that we had keys made so that we would be able to enter our clinic room at our own convenience. Mrs. Wilson immediately had new locks put on the doors so that we were unable to get into the building without hunting up the janitor.[92]

Such antipathy may help to explain why Pomeroy's practice was not widely followed. There is no evidence that either the city clinics or the two county institutions employed Spanish-speaking staff in any capacity.[93] Summarizing his interview with a Mexican immigrant, an anthropologist wrote that the man's wife "has never gone to the county hospital to give birth to a child. He is afraid that they will treat her badly which he has heard they do with the sick who can't make themselves understood with the doctors and nurses."[94] Because TB patients remained in institutions for months and sometimes years, we can easily imagine that those who spoke no English would have been extremely reluctant to apply for admission.

Nevertheless, the major charge against Mexican tuberculosis patients was the same one leveled against other poor people with the disease: rather than rejecting care, they used excessive amounts and thus overwhelmed government budgets. In the mid-1920s, the California State Board of Health published two widely circulated reports, which helped to shape the anti-Mexican discourse during the subsequent decade and a half. The first, *A Statistical Study of Sickness among the Mexicans in the Los Angeles County Hospital, from July 1, 1922 to June 30, 1924*, appeared in 1925.[95] It consisted largely of a series of statistical tables showing that between 1922 and 1924, Mexicans spent a total of 122,033 days in the hospital, at a cost to the county of $328,075. Tuberculosis represented 14 percent of all admissions; the cost to the county of care for Mexicans with tuberculosis was $75,141.[96] The following year, the State Board of Health published a second study, entitled *Summary of Mexican Cases Where Tuberculosis Is a Problem*.[97] The statistical tables had been compiled by R. R. Miller, the superintendent of the Outdoor Relief Division of the Los Angeles County Department of Charities. Those tables indicated that 374 Mexican families in Los Angeles "where tuberculosis is a problem" received county relief and/or state aid. (The Mothers Pension Act of 1921 provided $10 a month for children whose fathers could not work because of tuberculosis.) The annual expenditure for the 374 families was $154,851.60; the total amount spent to date was $292,406.54.

The timing of the two reports helps us understand their import. Both appeared shortly after the passage of the Immigration Act of 1924, which instituted numerical quotas for European immigrants.[98] In the introduction to the *Statistical Study*, Edythe Tate-Thompson, the director of the Bureau of Tuberculosis, noted that the act "does not help California" because it failed to impose a quota for Mexicans. The act did, however, profoundly alter the status of Mexicans, by precipitating the passage of various measures to tighten the border between Mexico and America and penalize those who entered unofficially.[99] Deportations rose from 1,751 in 1925 to over 15,000 in 1929, more than an eightfold increase.[100]

Tate-Thompson's introduction noted that deportation offered one remedy to the problems imposed by Mexicans with tuberculosis, suggesting that she endorsed those removals. But she also insisted that deportation provided inadequate protection because of the length and porosity of the border. One example highlighted the danger of unrestricted immigration:

Last year an aged Mexican in the last stages of tuberculosis came across the border unattended and of course unexamined, and a few hours later he was sent to the already overcrowded ward of the tuberculosis hospital. He was put to bed and on the second day decided he would not stay in bed in spite of a fever of 104 degrees, so he left the hospital and later was picked up on the street again and returned. . . . While the patient was waiting to be readmitted, he died. The incident was most unfortunate, the hospital was blamed, yet the episode of dying people entering this country is not unusual.[101]

Tate-Thompson's primary proposal was the one Pomeroy had recommended in 1917: the federal government should exercise greater control over the entire length of the border with Mexico.

Tate-Thompson's emphasis on tubercular Mexicans as economic burdens rather than as disease carriers also was reasonable within the context of growing agitation for an extension of the Immigration Act to people from the Western Hemisphere. To be sure, it was easier to quantify the costs of hospital days and monetary relief than to estimate the extent or rapidity of the spread of germs. Moreover, it was common to note that tuberculosis was a communicable, not a contagious, disease. And, as Tate-Thompson later remarked, Mexicans interacted with whites relatively infrequently.[102] Nevertheless, Tate-Thompson undoubtedly was aware that the primary argument for restricting immigration was that the costs inflicted by Mexican workers far outweighed the benefits they conferred. As the Order of Native Sons of the Golden West wrote in 1927, "It is evident that, unless an end is put to the influx of Mexicans, this country will have merely substituted a low-grade Westerner for a European immigrant, with a new race problem thrown in. . . . The effect of this Mexican influx on the already over-burdened taxpayer should be considered. Los Angeles County . . . is the dumping ground for poverty-stricken Mexicans."[103] Concerns about economic dependency had long dominated immigration policy; the main reason immigration authorities categorized tuberculosis as an "excludable condition" was not fear of the germs victims spread but rather the belief that they were "likely to become a public charge."[104] We have seen that similar considerations underlay the campaign to stem the tide of invalids into Southern California.

Tate-Thompson probably realized that her introduction did not express the opinions of all health officers. Some undoubtedly had close ties to employers. Pomeroy may have been especially loath to antagonize those who established the company towns where he situated health centers. Tate-Thompson, however, tarred all employers with the same brush, stating that her primary goal was to rebut their assertion that Mexicans represented a "cheap" form of labor and that the border therefore should be left open.[105] Her statistics, she claimed, demonstrated that employers' calculations ignored the enormous expenses Mexicans imposed on the state.

Tate-Thompson's contention that Mexicans imported tuberculosis also was somewhat controversial. After reporting fifty-nine tuberculosis deaths among

Mexicans in 1916, Pomeroy wrote that they "contracted the disease for the most part in California."[106] Governor Young's "Mexican Fact-Finding Committee" would reach a similar conclusion in 1930. Relying on 1926 charity cases in Los Angeles County, the report noted that seven-eighths of the heads of Mexican families with tuberculosis had been born in Mexico. Four-fifths, however, had lived in the United States more than five years; such data indicated to the committee that infection had occurred here.[107] Indeed, the belief that tuberculosis was imported contradicted the assertion that Mexican susceptibility resulted from lack of exposure. Tate-Thompson's one piece of evidence was highly improbable (an elderly migrant crossing the border and then traveling to Los Angeles in the final stages of disease). In 1928, she again suggested such cases were common: "There is often the case of the man who has been brought in as part of a construction gang and who has had a hemorrhage and been taken off at the first stop in California, and who perhaps lived only a few days."[108] The typical Mexican who crossed the border, she implied, was not the healthy worker employers sought but rather the invalid who had no productive capacity and consumed scarce public resources.

After publishing the two reports, Tate-Thompson ensured that they figured prominently in the growing campaign to extend the quota system. In January 1928 she mailed several copies of both to Albert Johnson, urging him to distribute them to members of the House Immigration Committee, which he chaired.[109] On February 1, 1930, she wrote again, sending him "some information that will show what Mexicans are costing certain sections of the state."[110] Two weeks later, she congratulated Johnson "on the splendid fight that you have made so successfully on the quota" and indicated that she would be "glad" to "furnish any additional information."[111]

Despite differences between Tate-Thompson and other officials, they rallied to the cause of restriction. A sociologist at the University of Southern California noted in 1934 that "social and public health workers" were an important group demanding extension of the quota.[112] Many claimed special expertise about Mexicans. Sixty-one public health nurses and social workers in Los Angeles signed a petition stating that they "have extensive and intimate knowledge of our foreign born population" and "believe in immigration restriction, as necessary to maintain the unity and safety of our country."[113] A physician at the Los Angeles County Department of Health East Side Health Center wrote to Johnson on behalf of a group of doctors and dentists who "are in close touch with the situation on the east side of Los Angeles (Belvedere and Maravilla Park) which is rapidly becoming intolerable to American tax payers" and who "feel especially qualified to speak on the subject."[114]

State and local officials also were important players in the hearings organized by Representative John C. Box of Texas on the bill to limit Mexican immigration. Pomeroy, for example, stated, "Unless the tubercular and venereal Mexican is cared for through the public health department he is likely to become a public health problem of sufficient size to affect the general public health."[115] Others testifying at the hearings portrayed Mexicans as economic burdens, pointing over and over to statistics from the two reports Tate-Thompson had circulated so effectively throughout the country.[116]

In short, health officials aggressively promoted the politics of exclusion in Los Angeles. At a time when elites were committed to establishing an exclusively Anglo-Saxon society, state and local authorities probably assumed that they could make a convincing case for adequate resources only by promising to safeguard the health of the white majority. If officials mirrored prevailing attitudes and responded to the particular context in which they operated, however, they also made unique contributions. By establishing separate clinics for Mexicans and whites, officials expanded patterns of segregation. They also added grist to the nativist mill when they portrayed Mexicans as economic burdens. And by exploiting white fears, officials may have helped to intensify them. Because public health authorities spoke with the voice of scientific authority, their portrayal of Mexicans as dangerous and burdensome carried special weight.[117]

And yet science could challenge popular prejudices as well as bolster them. In 1931 Emil Bogen, the medical director of Olive View Sanatorium, published a report disputing the belief that Mexicans had a racial susceptibility to tuberculosis. His autopsy study found "several instances of carcinoma of the lungs and other non-tuberculous conditions" which had "been clinically considered tuberculous"; this suggested to Bogen that "the cited high tuberculosis rates among the Mexicans may be due in part to oftener missed diagnoses of other conditions."[118] Moreover, at admission Mexicans tended to have more advanced disease than whites. Bogen concluded that "the greatest discrepancy between the death-rates from tuberculosis in patients of different nationalities, in this institution at least, arises from the fact that some groups are admitted early in the disease, and others later, and bears little relationship to any innate differences in their reaction to the infection after it has reached a certain stage."[119]

Had Bogen published his study at another time, it might have helped to counter some of the anti-Mexican discourse. Instead, as the shadow of the Great Depression descended on Los Angeles, health authorities increasingly sought to demonize Mexicans to justify a campaign of expulsion. Surviving records give no indication that any official noted the significance of Bogen's finding.

Chapter 5

Slashing Services in the Great Depression

Ever anxious to portray Los Angeles as uniquely favored, both the boosters and the local press initially claimed that the metropolis was exempt from the worst ravages of the Great Depression. By late 1931, however, few could deny that the cataclysm had struck Los Angeles as swiftly and severely as the rest of the country. Manufacturing output had dropped by 38 percent while business failures and unemployment had soared.[1]

But if the boosters no longer could ignore the depression, they could try to use it to stimulate tourism. The publicity literature urged easterners beset by financial stress to travel to the land of peace and tranquility. Advertisements in national magazines featured visitors relaxing by pools and oceans or strolling along picturesque mountain trails.[2] Seeking to highlight the healing qualities of the region, the two major booster organizations, the All-Year Club and the Chamber of Commerce, investigated the possibility of reopening some of the state's mineral springs.[3]

The tensions that had simmered for many years between health and welfare officers and the boosters now exploded. As poverty-stricken migrants flowed into the metropolis looking for work, officials charged the publicists with encouraging the wrong kind of migration. In response, the boosters reminded the public about the exclusivity of the promotional campaign. Rather than appealing to the unemployed from other states, publicists sought to develop "desirable tourist travel," consisting solely of "the more intelligent and substantial type of citizen." The All-Year Club pointed out that it advertised only in "the best magazines," which "reach the top layers of buying power nationally."[4] In 1934, the organization made plans to direct a special campaign to "retired individuals possessing independent incomes."[5]

Under pressure from the County Board of Supervisors, the chamber and All-Year Club agreed to append legends such as the following to all literature: "WARNING! While attractions for tourists are unlimited, please advise anyone seeking employment not to come to Southern California."[6] But those messages failed to mollify everyone. After interviewing an impoverished Texan woman whose husband and oldest son were in the hospital with tuberculosis, Edythe Tate- Thompson, the director of the State Bureau of Tuberculosis, remarked:

> I certainly would like to pass [her] story on to the Chambers of Commerce in this state as her reply, after . . . I tried to make her see that she ought to be ashamed when so much had been given her, was that with all the advertising that was done about California, that the least they could do, when people came in here, was to do better by them. This may be the key to the reason why the state has been deluged with migratory people. The Chambers of Commerce led them to believe that this is the "Promised Land"; that they could get anything when they got here.[7]

Conflicts about funding also erupted. For many years, the major booster organizations had received sizeable annual contributions from the Board of Supervisors. As the financial crisis deepened, however, some observers argued that the appropriations could better be spent on the county hospital or local relief programs.[8] Records of the All-Year Club indicate that between 1930–31 and 1931–32, its county funding dropped by half (from $500,000 to $250,000). By 1935–36, the appropriation had fallen to $155,000; after that it slowly rose, reaching $239,470 in 1936–37.[9] The organization's leaders continually asserted they helped to restore the Southern California economy by encouraging tourism, but that argument sounded somewhat hollow to many officials, trying to address overwhelming needs with dwindling resources.

Although gaps in the records make it impossible to gauge the full extent of the devastation wrought by the crisis, surviving documents amply demonstrate that it severely affected all segments of the nascent tuberculosis control program. In 1933 Tate-Thompson noted that the clinics operated by the City Department of Health were "turning an average of forty patients away daily."[10] Three years later, Director George Parish complained, "The daily clinics are overrun with people. It is not an uncommon practice to close the day's work an hour or two after the regular closing time with twenty-five or thirty people still waiting to be treated. These poor people are told to go home and come back in a day or two. This practice is unfair to them, most of whom are financially embarrassed, and in many instances, have spent their last dime to get here."[11] Many patients who gained admission received substandard care. In 1931, Dr. Harry

Cohn, the director of the Division of Tuberculosis, declared, "This community stands indicted until a properly equipped X-ray laboratory is given to this Department."[12] Nevertheless, it was not until 1936 that he was able to announce, "With the installation of X-ray equipment, during the coming year, the Tuberculosis Division will . . . no longer be required to apologize for the type of service rendered."[13] Within three years, however, the new machines had become inadequate. In 1939, Cohn complained, "The total clinic attendance has increased over four thousand during the past year. This has involved, in addition to the increased load on the medical personnel, unusual demands upon the X-ray service, which is limited by deficiency in appropriation. It is obvious that early case finding is the keynote in economic saving and in the opportunities for recovery."[14]

County programs also suffered. One of the first state legislative responses to the depression was to lengthen residence requirements. Before 1931, counties had been responsible for providing relief to all needy people who had lived in the state for one year and the county for three months. After that date, county obligations were restricted to people who had lived in the state for three years and in the county for one. Although the new law did not apply to the programs under the purview of the Department of Health, the change greatly restricted access to the two institutions operated by the Department of Charities (Olive View Sanatorium and L.A. General Hospital).[15]

Funding cutbacks affected those facilities in other ways. The state subsidy for Olive View patients remained constant throughout the 1930s,[16] but county appropriations plummeted. The daily cost per patient thus dropped from $3.29 in 1930–31 to $1.93 in 1934–45.[17] The cuts fell most heavily on the nursing staff. In 1934, a local group of businesswomen complained to the Board of Supervisors that 115 graduate nurses received "in addition to the regular salary cuts, a demotion to the rank of untrained attendants."[18] After visiting the sanatorium two years later, Tate-Thompson wrote, "The economy campaign that has gone on for the past two and a half years has reduced the nursing force to the point where there has been so few night nurses on duty that some buildings were left entirely without nurses or one nurse would have charge of as many as three buildings and have to walk a hundred yards between the buildings. Recently two girls died in a building where there was no nurse."[19]

And large numbers of patients who previously would have found beds at Olive View instead were relegated to private rest homes. Scattered throughout the county, these facilities contracted with the Department of Charities to provide care. The placements rarely pleased patients. One reason was that most facilities were even more remote than Olive View. Tate-Thompson noted that many people worried about being sent "too far from their families."[20] Emilia Castañeda de Valenciana later described the trip she took from Belvedere to a rest home in the San Fernando Valley to see her mother: "I remember us traveling by bus, which made me car sick every time we used to go to visit her. . . . Maybe it was the fumes of the bus or something that made me become ill. By the time I used to get there, I was half sick from the bus trip."[21]

In addition, as officials often acknowledged, the quality of rest-home care was seriously deficient. Tate-Thompson often told horror stories. In January 1933, she visited "a rest home located on a hill with fifty-seven steep steps to climb to reach the house. . . . I wondered how patients managed after being brought there in an ambulance." The same month she reported the death of "a woman from exposure because the pipes had frozen in the barn where she was being housed, so she was obliged to leave the building and walk over into another building to a toilet. She had a hemorrhage." Other patients "went into the garbage cans for catsup and vinegar bottles, trying to fill those with hot water."[22] In February Tate-Thompson inspected a "horrible place" in Newhall. "It was a warm day, 'rest hour,' gas furnaces on full blast, dirty windows closed so that the air was fetid." A county health department survey revealed "nests of mice, mites, rats and a variety of insects in the kitchen."[23]

Although county officials initially had assumed the rest homes would serve a predominantly convalescent clientele, many residents were very sick. After visiting a facility in 1933, Tate-Thompson reported that "some extremely ill patients have been sent from the General Hospital. In fact, one . . . was sent from the General Hospital in almost a dying condition."[24] In 1936–37, more than three-quarters of rest-home residents were classified as "far advanced."[25] Physician visits, however, were few and far between. In June 1934, Tate-Thompson wrote, "Recently in a place for boys, a boy began hemorrhaging with a fever of 103. The caretaker, a practical nurse, tried the usual procedure of ice bags and salt. She had no ice so she decided a tepid bath was indicated, so the boy was carried in and placed in the bath. His temperature came down but the bleeding continued—much to the woman's surprise. Finally a physician, fifteen miles away was sent for. I suppose he was as surprised as I was that, with the patient almost bleeding to death, he had not died from such treatment."[26]

Despite the closure of a few of the worst facilities in 1934, criticisms continued to mount. In 1936, Everett J. Gray, the Olive View superintendent, wrote, "Many complaints that have been received from patients in rest homes are based on the lack of medical attention they receive." Gray had "but 3½ doctors responsible for this work, resulting in a ratio of one doctor to two hundred fifty patients." With the rest homes "scattered over an area of 2,000 square miles," the doctors were compelled to "spend considerable of their time in traveling from one place to another."[27] Four years later Tate-Thompson found three facilities "too crowded either from the standpoint of health or for safety from the standpoint of a fire hazard. " Because the "three feet necessary between the beds" did not exist, the "possibilities for reinfection" were "very great."[28] Nevertheless, the number of rest homes grew steadily during the 1930s; by the end of the decade, twenty facilities served approximately thousand patients (nearly the same number as in Olive View).[29]

One place where quality of care did improve was in the county hospital. A 1923 bond issue had raised funds for a new building, and an imposing, twenty-story structure finally opened on State Street in April 1934. "The new hospital seemed very magnificent to those who had worked in the old hospital," one historian writes. "The wards were no longer crowded with 50 to 60 patients, as they were in the past. . . . The wards were uncrowded and the hospital was clean and new, all of which provided a welcome change from the old hospital."[30] Unfortunately, tuberculosis patients were not among the chief beneficiaries. Tate-Thompson insisted that they be transferred not to the new facility but rather to the building that had previously served as the surgical unit. As she explained, "It would appear that in the new hospital, they are having a great deal of difficulty in discharging patients, as they are more comfortable than they ever have been in their lives." With "fewer comforts," the "chances are that their stay would not be quite as long as it would be if their convalescing were done in the new building."[31] In January 1935 Tate-Thompson noted that the hospital was so "packed" that some tuberculosis patients had to be moved to the new building.[32] By that date, however, many people had difficulty gaining access to any part of the hospital. "Daily physicians call up," she wrote, "objecting to the long, long delay for admission."[33]

Two assaults by the medical profession damaged the clinics operated by the Department of Health. Ever since the establishment of dispensaries in major eastern cities in the late eighteenth century, doctors had fought the delivery of free or low-cost medical care to the poor. The editor of the *Medical Record*, Dr. G. Shrady, wrote, "It is simply not true that poor people suffer for want of skilled medical attendance. On the contrary, they obtain vastly more than they have a right to expect. . . . Vast sums of money are wasted yearly on worthless and undeserving persons."[34] Such complaints grew especially vehement after the stock market crash as patients unable to afford the fees private physicians charged increasingly abandoned their offices for public clinics. Under the auspices of the American Medical Association, the newly established Physicians' Public Health League campaigned for the restriction of public health activities.[35]

Notable for offering curative as well as preventive care, the health centers operated by the County Department of Health were a prime target for attack.

In 1931, the league, in conjunction with the Los Angeles County Medical Association (LACMA), demanded that the centers cease furnishing medical care to patients whose diseases did not threaten public health.[36] We can surmise why Department of Health director John L. Pomeroy offered no resistance. He had long complained about the need to provide care for noncommunicable diseases, and one response to budget cutbacks had been to ask the Department of Charities to help defray the cost.[37] When that department refused, the matter was submitted to the county counsel, who ruled that Pomeroy was "authorized only to treat cases involving contagious diseases which are a menace to the public health." His request for reimbursement from the charities department was denied because he should have "nothing to do with the work of the county in the care of the sick where no question of public health is involved."[38]

The changes LACMA requested went into effect early in 1932. Health department clinics continued to provide treatment for two afflictions that had potential to endanger the public health—venereal disease and tuberculosis. Care for all other diseases was transferred to the out-patient clinic at the county hospital (operated by the Department of Charities).[39] The result was a significant decline in access. Patients from outlying areas in the county had to travel dozens of miles to downtown Los Angeles for care. In addition, because the residence requirements of the charities department were far more rigid than those of the health department, many people lost eligibility.[40]

To some extent, that episode demonstrates the privileged status of people with TB. At a time when other indigent patients faced new barriers to care, the access of tuberculosis sufferers remained unaltered. But special treatment came at a high cost. Tuberculosis was now firmly linked with venereal disease, an even more stigmatized affliction. And once again TB patients were deemed eligible for care only because their germs threatened the broader society, not because their lives had intrinsic value.

That focus became still more pronounced when LACMA launched a second major assault in 1933, demanding that county health centers discontinue all preventive services, including tuberculosis screening and diagnosis. That attack struck at the heart of Pomeroy's authority, and he mounted a strong defense, galvanizing support from public health officials throughout the nation. As he wrote to the Board of Supervisors, the "control of communicable diseases" was a "function of the police power of the health officer and not a charitable function of the county"; indeed, it was "by far the most important major function of the health department and to the people." Furthermore, the Department of Charities had authority to care only for people who qualified under the state residence law. Its services thus excluded "hundreds of persons . . . afflicted annually with infectious diseases."[41]

Pomeroy attached a memo from Zdenka Buben, chief of the Division of Medical Social Service, providing several examples of such persons. One was a forty-nine-year-old man who lived with his wife and child, as well as his wife's married son and the son's ten-year-old child. The entire family was "a very unintelligent type." The patient's "personal habits" were "detrimental to [the] health of family and community." Buben concluded that "considerable damage could be done were it not possible to arrange medical and nursing supervision in the Health Department pending completion of the social plan for the family."[42]

Pomeroy also supported his case by enclosing the thirty-three letters he had received from the national public health community. "I cannot believe," wrote Kendall Emerson, executive secretary of the American Public Health Association, "that the medical profession would insist on the point that x-ray equipment should not be permitted in a diagnostic clinic for tuberculosis, since it is admitted in any informed medical circle that such clinic for tuberculosis without x-ray equipment has no right to be in operation."[43] Haven Emerson wrote from Columbia University College of Physicians and Surgeons, "It is unthinkable that the clinic management of tuberculosis should pass out of the hands of the health department, until welfare and hospital services are under a much higher quality of medical direction with a keen sense of responsibility to discover and eliminate infection."[44] Some officials disputed the motives of the medical association. "It seems to me deplorable," wrote Graham A. Laing, professor of economics from the California Institute of Technology, "that there should be such a general attempt to treat the health of the public as a matter for purely commercial treatment by practicing physicians."[45] Others noted that the doctors' actions were part of a national campaign to undermine public health. "I am not surprised to hear that the Los Angeles County Medical Society is attempting to stop most of the public health work in your county," wrote John P. Koehler, Milwaukee's commissioner of health. "I went through this same battle about a year ago."[46]

This time Pomeroy ultimately prevailed. Although the records do not indicate why the board denied LACMA's request, they indicate that TB screening and diagnosis remained under the control of the Department of Health. Tubercular patients undoubtedly benefited—though only at the price of being identified more closely than ever with dangerous germs.

If TB patients continued to be singled out for special care by the county health department, they received no benefit from the New Deal programs established after President Roosevelt's 1932 election. Seeking to restore the dignity of workers thrust out of their jobs by the depression, those programs sharpened the traditional welfare distinction between the able-bodied and non-able-bodied. Sick and disabled people were considered "the naturally dependent" and thus remained the responsibility of local programs.[47] Although staff often clashed about whether specific applicants were "employable" or "nonemployable," a tuberculosis label automatically settled the issue.[48] Even patients well enough to hold part-time or "light" jobs were deemed ineligible for assistance from the State Emergency Relief Administration, the State Relief Administration, and the Works Progress Administration.

People with tuberculosis did continue to qualify for relief from the Los Angeles County Department of Charities. The new residence requirement, however, meant that all newcomers were disqualified. And funding cutbacks made the assistance far less attractive to eligible clients. The wait to file applications at local offices often lasted most of the day.[49] Even worse, the average monthly family allowance fell from an average of $21.55 per family in 1928–29 to $8.83 in 1931–32, a 59 percent drop.[50] While county officials invoked the familiar argument that larger stipends would attract the unworthy, public health leaders repeatedly complained that tubercular clients could not afford the living arrangements doctors recommended.[51] (Not surprisingly, the depression intensified conflicts between different local agencies, each seeking to blame the other for the sharp rise in TB rates.) The County Department of Charities occasionally paid extra rent for tuberculosis patients or moved them to larger and brighter apartments; the great majority, however, remained in poorly ventilated and overcrowded accommodations.[52]

Because TB patients were advised to eat large quantities of eggs, milk, and meat, the miserly food budgets provoked even greater consternation. In 1931, Harry Cohn, director of the City Division of Tuberculosis, wrote to the Board of Supervisors that examinations of tuberculosis patients discharged from Olive View indicated a "reactivation of their disease," caused "in most instances" by "improper nutrition." "Unless plans are formulated by the proper agencies for satisfactory relief of these tuberculous sick," he warned, "many of these patients, who could be self supporting, if relief were continued for a short period of time after discharge from the sanatorium, will become sick and dependent."[53] According to Tate-Thompson, the cutbacks in food budgets ultimately resulted in economic inefficiencies: "One cannot judge the Welfare Department too harshly because they have carried a load that, unless one saw it in operation, would seem almost impossible, but no money is being saved . . . when a patient who has had a long period of care at Olive View, returns home to live on such a limited budget that in a few months everything they have gained at Olive View has been lost."[54] A "Committee on Tuberculosis" chaired by Dr. Francis M. Pottenger reported to the Department of Charities in August 1934:

> People who have a chronic illness, such as tuberculosis, suffer from lack of appetite and digestive disturbances and not infrequently show inability to eat certain types of foods. . . . Hence, a standard grocery package which might be of sufficient food value for a healthy individual, might not be suitable for a patient with active or recently arrested tuberculosis. We believe that it would be economical for the county to give them a diet that would maintain them in a proper state of nutrition, even at a greater per capita cost.[55]

Tate-Thompson noted that special allotments of meat, eggs, and milk continued to be available, but only when "Oked by the clinic physician." "Very often," however, tuberculosis patients were "too ill to get to the clinic. It is a terrible situation."[56]

In August 1938, a group of nutritionists hired by the board of supervisors to assess the "county indigent budget" concluded that it provided only "an emergency diet, definitely below any acceptable dietary standard" and recommended a 54 percent increase.[57] Nevertheless, the county reduced the allowance still further the following month.[58] In December, Tate-Thompson wrote, "Many families come to the office complaining that they are not getting enough to eat, and I would be inclined to think there must be some truth in their complaints."[59]

Not all patients suffered equally from the depression-era budget cutbacks. Because the financial crisis exaggerated fears and antipathies, a tuberculosis diagnosis began to acquire a far more ominous meaning for anyone whom elite Los Angelenos considered an outsider. The receipt of either financial assistance or health services started to seem even more illegitimate than ever. And exclusion increasingly expanded to mean not only preventing unwanted social groups from entering the metropolis, but also confining them in special institutions and transporting them back to their homes.

Chapter 6

Expelling Mexicans and Filipinos

The most searing event in the early life of Mary Helen Ponce, the daughter of Mexican immigrants in the San Fernando Valley, was the death of her brother Rito. Rito had joined the Civilian Conservation Corps as a teenager in the late 1930s but returned home when he was diagnosed with tuberculosis and died just before the outbreak of World War II. Mary Helen had only fleeting memories of him—his sadness, his blue-green eyes, the gentle touch of his thin fingers when he combed her tangled hair, and the blue cotton pajamas he wore as a patient at Olive View Sanatorium. But she vividly remembered the church funeral and the walk home with her mother. "When the big black hearse went by, my mother wavered in her step, then stopped. She stood deathly still until the hearse had passed, then slowly pulled back her hat veil. 'Adios hijo mio.' "[1]

Rito was the second of the Ponce children to succumb to tuberculosis. Born in Mexico and arriving in Los Angeles as an infant, Rosalie, too, had spent her last years at Olive View. Mary Helen knew her sister only from the photograph which portrayed a serious thirteen-year-old; she died at eighteen, when Mary Helen was three months old. Their mother "never recovered" from Rosalie's death; the loss of a second child was even more devastating.[2]

In official accounts, Rito and Rosalie appear as statistics documenting the excessive burdens Mexicans imposed on government coffers. The 1930 report of Governor C. C. Young's "Mexican Fact-Finding Committee" claimed that the cost of treating Mexicans in Los Angeles General Hospital had increased "more than a third" since 1925.[3] As government funding for tuberculosis care plummeted during the depression, such an expense—combined with that of caring for Mexicans in Olive View and in both city and county clinics—began to seem even more indefensible than before.

The County Department of Health repeatedly focused on the high Mexican tuberculosis rate. The 1936–37 report read, "Attention must be drawn to the fact that Mexicans make up 22.5 per cent of the cases, which shows that the disease is greatly out of the proportion to their percentage of the population, which is approximately 10 per cent."[4] The following year the department wrote, "Attention . . . is again directed to the tremendous burden on this County through certain problems among the Mexicans. Most noteworthy is the situation on tuberculosis. For the State of California as a whole, while the Mexican makes up only 6½ per cent of the total population, 21½ per cent of the deaths from tuberculosis occur among this group."[5]

Because many private physicians failed to report tuberculosis cases and deaths in deference to patient wishes, those statistics can easily be disputed. Too poor to consult private physicians, many Mexicans enrolled in public clinics and thus may have been especially likely to be labeled tubercular in official reports. Difficulties estimating the size of the Mexican population compounded the problem.[6] And preconceptions about Mexicans as tubercular appear to have inflated the statistics, which then were used to prove the point. Mary Helen Ponce recalled that school nurses assumed that every undernourished Mexican child suffered from tuberculosis.[7] From the time the county instituted school screening programs in the early 1930s, Mexican children were especially likely to be the focus. The 1937–38 County Health Department report noted that elementary-school screening occurred only in districts "abounding in tuberculosis or such as were attended largely by racial or economic groups especially subject to the disease"; that same year, the department "started testing all Mexican infants under one year coming to our Baby Welfare Clinics, hoping that the reactors in this group will lead us to yet undetected cases."[8] Emil Bogen's autopsy report of Olive View patients suggests that preconceptions may have influenced the process of diagnosis as well as the target of screening. As we recall, he concluded that "the cited high tuberculosis rates among the Mexicans may be due in part to oftener missed diagnoses of other conditions."[9]

The 1937–38 report of the Department of Health also contained the results of two in-depth studies of tuberculosis among Mexicans. Director John L. Pomeroy noted that the first had been conducted "under my orders" in "a Mexican settlement known as Maravilla Park." In April 1937 the chest clinic serving that three-mile area had "118 cases of active tuberculosis," "196 arrested cases," and another "196 showing infection or positive tuberculin test." According to Pomeroy, the study demonstrated the consequences of poor housing. Although "the average family consisted of 5.2 persons," the "majority of houses consisted of less than 4 rooms." Most homes were "of flimsy construction of food, many not weather-proofed, commonly infested with pests and bugs, harboring filth throughout." Floors "frequently" were "in poor repair."[10] Pomeroy concluded, "It is impossible to accomplish proper results with our public health staff when the basic foundation, adequate housing, is lacking."[11]

Because most experts viewed tuberculosis as a "house disease," Pomeroy's focus made good sense.[12] Moreover, because many Maravilla Park residents relied on county relief, he could blame the Department of Charities for providing such paltry allowances that recipients could not afford better accommodations. Diverting attention from conditions over which he had jurisdiction (such as sanitation or the quality of clinic or public health nursing care), Pomeroy stressed that the "Los Angeles County Charities Department is responsible for the housing conditions of over half of these families."[13] Nevertheless, Pomeroy did not completely absolve the residents themselves. The phrase "harboring filth" implicated housewives as well as landlords and the Department of Charities. He noted that overcrowding stemmed not only from the small size of the dwellings but also from the "large families" Mexicans produced. The resistance of Mexicans to institutionalization increased the likelihood that they would spread germs to family and friends. ("Out of 42 patients of active tuberculosis in need of placement in sanatoria, 22 refused to go.")[14] And once again he emphasized the special vulnerability of Mexican bodies. Despite the absence of any comparative data, Pomeroy asserted that high tuberculosis rates among children indicated "that in Mexican families the infection takes place earlier and more intensively than among the population in general."[15]

Pomeroy's summary of the second study read:

> A most notable examination of how tuberculosis can spread among the family group is herewith given. The original settler of a certain family came from Mexico in 1885. Of 96 individuals known to the Health Department descended from this person, among some 20 families there have been during the past seven year period, 5 deaths from tuberculosis, 8 active cases, 5 with the childhood type, 2 arrested adult type, 7 arrested childhood type and <u>48 showed by tuberculin test that they are infected at the present time but as yet have no active demonstrable lesions by x-ray</u>. [Underlined in original][16]

This study was conducted in conjunction with the Department of Charities, which also reported the results. According to that department's account, the disease had been traced "to a couple entering this country from Mexico." By omitting the entry date of the first "settler" (fifty-three years earlier) and the fact that most family members thus had been born in the United States and contracted tuberculosis here, the report helped to fuel fears about immigrants introducing disease into the metropolis. The report also stated that "the majority" of descendants were "afflicted with tuberculosis," ignoring the distinction between infection and active disease.[17] According to the Department of Health, nearly half the family members had tested positive on the tuberculin test, but only a small minority had discernible symptoms.

Other incendiary and misleading information appeared in the monthly reports of Edythe Tate-Thompson, the director of the Bureau of Tuberculosis. Her primary concern was to demonstrate that, contrary to grower claims, Mexicans represented an unacceptably expensive labor force throughout the state. Because tuberculosis struck large numbers of Orange County Mexicans, "the entire Mexican population" would "ultimately be unloaded on the taxpayers of the County."[18] San Bernardino County "had the highest death rate in the United States" as a result of the "large numbers of Mexican laborers brought in who very quickly become centers of infection to large groups of both Americans and Mexicans." In both Riverside and San Bernardino, residents had "over a long period of years . . . grown accustomed to the cough of the Mexican consumptive and have assumed an attitude that they were transients or casual laborers not worthy of mention socially, but from the standpoint of the epidemiology of the disease they are very much worth while." As in her introduction to the 1925 *Statistical Study of Sickness among the Mexicans in the Los Angeles County Hospital*, Tate-Thompson used personal observation to bolster official data: "Once I was in the tuberculosis pavilion when a carload of Mexicans were brought in to work. It was discovered [that] three of them were dying with tuberculosis."[19]

Tate-Thompson's key grievance was that Mexicans overutilized expensive institutional services. Because "80 per cent" of the ninety-two tuberculosis beds in Orange County were occupied by Mexicans, "the white population . . . does not have an opportunity to get into the hospital."[20] In the city of San Bernardino, "99 percent of the children with active tuberculosis who have been in the children's pavilion are Mexicans."[21] In Los Angeles County, "patients especially Mexicans," were "left for years in the sanatoria."[22] In January 1933, Tate-Thompson "found one Mexican boy in Olive View since 1925."[23] She also visited the Fernandez family, "Mexicans of the lowest type."[24] The father "died of tuberculosis in 1924, the mother also has tuberculosis. Two children died with tuberculous meningitis. Jose was sent to Olive View in 1929 with tuberculosis of the spine. Rosa died at Olive View the same year. Apolona has tbc.

glands. Theresa and Juanita also went to Olive View in 1929. Finally, in 1932 the end of the year, Theresa was transferred to a Rest Home. Jose is still there though the doctor on August 13, 1932 requested he be removed."[25] In October 1933, Tate-Thompson estimated that "$12,500 had been spent giving hospital care to these subnormal Mexican children."[26]

Tate-Thompson's solution was that counties provide cheap, custodial care for many Mexicans, leaving costly hospital and sanatoria beds for worthier patients. In that way, she sought to reconcile the competing goals of protecting the white population and reducing health care expenditures. "At the request of the Superintendent of the Stanislaus County Hospital," Tate-Thompson wrote in May 1933, "I stopped at Modesto to discuss with him some plans for caring for patients. . . . There are many Mexicans and farm laborers in the advanced stages of tuberculosis who need isolation and care without having sanatorium care."[27] She had similar advice for Los Angeles. In October 1933 she visited the Santa Teresita Rest Home, operated by the Carmelite Sisters in Duarte. As usual, she stressed the poor quality of the rest home. Although the facililty contained "extremely ill patients," the doctor made "no regular calls" and left no instructions when he did. During an emergency the previous night, the nuns had been forced to summon a new doctor from a nearby town. He told Tate-Thompson that "he could not eat any lunch when he got back, for being so distressed in seeing a child so ill without a doctor on call." Nevertheless, she concluded that "many of the Mexican girls being sent to Olive View should be sent here instead."[28] After meeting with the rest home director in December, she commented, "Mexican patients transferred from Olive View object to the simple surroundings at the Sisters; and it would have been infinitely better judgment if the Placement Bureau had never sent Mexicans to Olive View."[29]

Elderly Mexican women were another group Tate-Thompson deemed undeserving of expensive institutional care. In December 1937 she accompanied a medical social worker in Belvedere on a visit to Mexican families with tuberculosis. "From the standpoint to the taxpayers," she concluded,

> I believe that a one story hospital of an inexpensive type of construction could be erected in Belvedere and be used to segregate or quarantine these Mexican cases. A check on the admissions into hospitals and rest homes in the county show that ultimately nearly all the members of these families receive care at public expense. I am doubtful if the old grandmothers, who frequently have been the source of contact as far as infection is concerned, should be given hospital care, but they do need to be removed from the families.[30]

By the time Tate-Thompson issued that report, two measures had reduced Mexican access to Olive View Sanatorium. The first was a 1930 law restricting the state subsidy to citizens. A 1940 study explained the reason for the change: "The number of cases in Mexican and oriental aliens which have a high rate of attack overtaxed the facilities available and the financial ability of the commonwealth."[31] Olive View statistics indicate that although Mexicans remained a high proportion of its patients, their composition changed dramatically. Most Mexicans in Los Angeles during the 1930s were noncitizens,[32] but the proportion of Mexican patients born in Mexico declined from 72 percent in 1927 to 30 percent in 1936.[33] (Because few Mexican immigrants became citizens, the place of birth could be considered a proxy measure for citizenship status.)

The second originated in local action. In 1932, the Los Angeles County Health Department and the County Department of Charities cooperated in establishing the Huntington Park Mexican Colony. The goal was to substitute a tuberculosis home care program for institutional services. The targeted area was "a small, poor, typical Mexican settlement" containing sixty-three families.[34] Authorities claimed that supervision of the entire household helped to contain disease and that Mexican patients were unusually homesick in Olive View. The primary benefits, however, were economic. The 1939 report of Violet Blanche Goldberg, a University of Southern California social work student, began, "The problem of institutional care for the Mexican tuberculosis cases has become a point of great interest to the taxpayer and the politician. Constant reference has been made to the problem of aliens without funds, who have been placed in sanatoria and hospitals, and announced a causative factor in the high taxes."[35] County officials noted that they saved $10,000 a year by keeping patients at home rather than sending them to Olive View.[36] Not surprisingly, Edythe Tate-Thompson was a strong proponent of the colony, urging that similar projects "be encouraged in all of the counties with a large Mexican population."[37]

Although surviving records do not enable us to evaluate whether prevailing prejudices affected the quality of care delivered to Mexicans who gained entry to Olive View, we do know that relatively few qualified for a major nonmedical program. In 1930, Tate-Thompson wrote that when she had appealed "for a separate appropriation to be used by the Rehabilitation Department of the State Board of Education for rehabilitation of some of the sanatoria patients and ex-patients," she "little reckoned on the far-reaching results." "Many a discouraged patient feeling rusty and out of touch with his former occupation finds the opportunity open to keep in touch with his job. . . . Day after day when making rounds . . . one sees in the wards typewriters on lapboards or bedside tables filled with textbooks that are being studied."[38] But at Olive View, whites were most likely to reap the program's benefits. A 1941 study reported, "Almost ninety per cent of the rehabilitated individuals were white. One Filipino, three Japanese and approximately twenty-five Mexicans were rehabilitated . . . . Since less than sixty per cent of the patients at Olive View Sanatorium are white, the rehabilitated group, with almost ninety per cent white, is a selected group as regards race."[39]

If some Mexicans encountered new barriers to care, others were forced to accept treatment. In January 1932, A. C. Price, the assistant superintendent of charities, asked Everett Mattoon, the county counsel, for authority to use the quarantine law to remove a Mexican man from the house he shared with his mother and his six children. Mattoon ruled that "the county health officer has the authority to compel forcible hospitalization of people afflicted with tuberculosis."[40] The number of people compelled to enter institutions under isolation orders grew slowly but steadily during the next few years, reaching 149 in 1939.[41]

A comment by Tate-Thompson suggests the measure was especially likely to affect Mexicans. After praising the operation of the new law in Los Angeles, she wrote, "I feel that because of the conjected [sic] areas in which they [Mexicans] live, and because of their lowered resistance, they become active cases much quicker than other people, and that whenever any person is found to be a spreader of tuberculosis, that the state and local health departments have a moral responsibility to see that the patient is removed from the home and the quarantine made rigid enough to impress the people away from them."[42] Pomeroy defended the unequal impact of the quarantine in various ways. "The Mexican frequently objects to going to institutions." "Forcible quarantine" was "necessary because most of these families are living under poor home conditions."[43] The study of the descendants of a Mexican immigrant couple showed "in a striking manner the way in which tuberculosis spreads in a family when the members who are sources of infection are not promptly and effectively isolated from other members."[44] And, finally, there was a compelling economic argument. Emphasizing the high rate of tuberculosis among Mexicans, Pomeroy commented, "When it is considered how small a per cent of the expense resulting from this situation is borne by Mexican people directly or by their taxes indirectly, we are justified in our close and sometimes arbitrary supervision of Mexicans with tuberculosis in a communicable state."[45]

Experts considered tubercular Mexicans burdensome not only because they used extensive health care but also because they appeared to receive a disproportionate share of monetary assistance. The influential Young Report repeated the conclusion of the 1926 *Summary of Mexican Cases Where Tuberculosis Is a*

Problem that Mexicans in Los Angleles represented "nearly two-fifths of all tuber-culosis cases in which county relief were granted." In addition, "nearly a fourth of all Mexican relief cases involved tuberculosis," compared to just one-tenth of all "non-Mexican cases."[46] Although Mexicans were the first to lose jobs after the stock market crash, many state and local relief efforts gave priority to whites; some excluded all noncitizens.[47] The Los Angeles County Department of Charities continued to provide relief to Mexicans but cut their allotments by 20 percent in 1933.[48] In a speech to directors of the department that year, Superintendent Earl Jensen stated, "Get it out of your mind that each family, Mexican, Chinese, and white should have the same average monthly require-ments." Mexican families did not need the same allotment for rent as whites:

> The matter of personal equation should enter into each case. A visitor should know that the needs of one family cannot be gauged by the needs of another. . . . I think you will agree with me that we are giving some of the Mexicans more than they ever had in their lives. . . . I don't care if the President of Mexico comes here and tells me I am discriminating, we must discriminate as between the man who lives as these Mexicans [have] in the past, as compared with another man who has always lived in a different environment.[49]

Jensen's primary rationale—that Mexicans spent less than whites on rent—was especially ironic in view of the repeated claim that high rates of tuberculosis stemmed partly from substandard, overcrowded housing. Other officials justi-fied the policy by arguing that Mexicans ate less expensive food, despite the widespread belief that poor diets abetted the onset of tuberculosis.[50]

This was not the first time that the Mexican standard of living had been used to justify lower stipends. A 1915 investigation of L.A. county outdoor relief by the Bureau of Efficiency and the State Board of Charities and Correction had urged that the "amount and kind of assistance" vary with "each case or type of case." For example, "adequate relief for an educated widow with four minor children who has lived at a standard, warranted by an income of $100 a month, presents a very different problem than that of the illiterate Mexican widow with an equally large family who has lived from hand to mouth and is possessed of no recognized standards of living."[51] For thirty years county offi-cials had rejected that recommendation, seeking to alter Mexican habits and practices and encouraging them aspire to "American" ways. Now financial exi-gency, combined with growing hostility toward Mexicans and a diminished commitment to assimilation, made a policy of differential stipends far more attractive.

Did the decisions of individual county staff also reflect the widespread anti-Mexican bias? Front-line bureaucrats in county welfare programs traditionally have enjoyed considerable discretion, and at least one incident suggests that was also the case in Los Angeles.[52] In October 1934, the United Council of Working Class Women, who defined themselves as "an elected committee of women representing Boyle Heights, City Terrace, Highland Park and Belvedere Women's Councils," wrote to the County Board of Supervisors about the "grievances of elderly and destitute women clients of Ferris Street Relief Station." Both were Mexican. One, "a very sick woman suffering from tuberculosis was left without care for weeks." When neighbors "went to the station to ask that [she] be taken care of, they were told to get out and not come any more, that it was none of their business." The council sent four women to protest, but the director of the station treated them "as rioters and criminals [and] called the county police who were rough and abusive." The council's letter demanded the dismissal of the director "as unfit and incompetent to administer relief to the people whom she does not regard to be human beings at all."[53]

The deportation and repatriation drives of the 1930s had by far the greatest impact on Mexicans with tuberculosis. Although several historians have described those campaigns, the role of that disease has received virtually no attention.[54] Concerned about the costs of supporting tubercular Mexicans, both state and local health authorities participated enthusiastically in both campaigns.

The deportation drive began shortly after the depression descended on Los Angeles. In 1930, Secretary of Labor William Doak stated that the best way to attack unemployment would be to expel "four hundred thousand illegal aliens."[55] By that date, the phrase "illegal aliens" had become another name for Mexicans; Doak concentrated his efforts on Southern California. He soon received help from Charles P. Visel, the director of the Los Angeles Citizens Committee on the Coordination of Unemployment Relief, a new organization of local civic leaders. In January 1931, Visel devised a plan to frighten Mexican immigrants into leaving the city without formal deportation hearings. He prepared an announcement of an impending deportation campaign, which he sent, in his words, to "all newspapers of Los Angeles, including especially the foreign language newspapers."[56] With Visel's support, immigration authorities conducted a series of highly publicized raids on Mexican communities. Agents went door to door, demanding that residents show proof of legal status and arresting those unable to do so. By February 21, 225 people had been apprehended.[57] Although that group included Chinese, Japanese, and whites, the supervisor of the Bureau of Immigration in Los Angeles wrote that "the Mexican element . . . predominates."[58] On February

26, federal agents surrounded the downtown plaza, detaining four hundred individuals, most of them Mexicans.[59]

Attempts to ferret out illegal immigrants must have been especially terrifying to Mexicans suffering from tuberculosis. By impoverishing Mexicans and forcing them to apply for relief, the disease also heightened their vulnerability to deportation. Moreover, the Supreme Court interpreted "entry" to mean the "last entry."[60] As one contemporary observer wrote, "Even after a few hours' visit in Mexico a health condition which has been present for many years while the person resided in the United States may make him excludable."[61] Because many Mexican immigrants in Los Angeles frequently traveled back and forth across the border,[62] that interpretation threatened them.

Although we have no way of determining whether health authorities endorsed the tactics employed by federal agents in Los Angeles, they traditionally had looked for aliens in public hospitals (along with asylums and jails).[63] In 1930, Tate-Thompson wrote, "Efforts have been made to deport Mexicans, or at least care for them only until the immigration authorities could deport them."[64] Two years later, the California Department of Public Health referred to its "Cooperation with the U.S. Immigration Service."[65] (Unfortunately, the department did not specify the nature of that cooperation.) In 1933, Tate-Thompson complained that the Fernandez family, whose many children resided in Olive View, "could have been deported years ago if any effort had been made to do so."[66]

Some evidence also suggests that just as welfare officials used the threat of deportation to encourage voluntary departure, so health authorities used that threat to compel compliance with medical regimes. According to a Master's thesis at the University of Southern California School of Social Work in 1939, the widespread fear of deportation proceedings helped to "force" recalcitrant Mexicans to accept institutional care.[67] In 1934, Tate-Thompson complained about a Mexican farm couple who were U.S. citizens. After noting the woman's refusal both to believe that her child had died from tuberculosis and to submit to an examination herself, Tate-Thompson concluded, "There is nothing as difficult to handle as an American-born Mexican . . . . They can and do defy everything and everybody."[68]

But the deportation campaign also may well have undermined public health goals. Reporting on the "first roundups of aliens," Watkins noted that many had gone "into hiding" and that they were "generally well informed as to the provisions of the immigration law and the conditions under which they may or may not be deported."[69] We can well imagine that long after the raids ceased, many Mexicans were unwilling to report symptoms of tuberculosis, undergo diagnostic examinations, or attend clinics. The executive secretary of the Los Angeles Tuberculosis and Health Association wrote in April 1934, "Patients who are not yet citizens of the United States and who have contracted tuberculosis often seek information regarding rules and regulations relative to deportation which might affect their care."[70] A social worker later recalled that breadwinners were extremely reluctant to accept institutionalization, knowing their departure would force other members of the family to rely on public assistance and thus increase the risk of deportation.[71] Mexicans must have been especially anxious to avoid home visits, which could reveal family members who wished to remain hidden and uncover such conditions as coresidence by unmarried couples, which might lead to deportation on grounds of moral turpitude.[72]

Repatriation differed from deportation in three ways.[73] First, returnees left voluntarily rather than after formal proceedings. (Mexicans on relief, however, frequently felt enormous pressure to depart).[74] Second, repatriation affected far more individuals. And third, it was organized by local rather than federal officials. In January 1931, the Los Angeles County Department of Charities asked

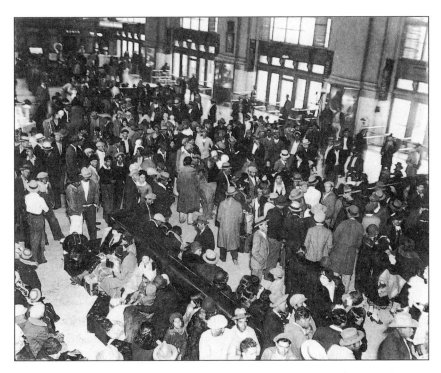

Figure 8.   Mexican families departing from Union Station, Los Angeles, 1932
Courtesy of Photograph Collection, Los Angeles Public Library.

the Board of Supervisors for funds to pay the rail fares of Mexicans to the border. The first repatriation train departed on March 23, 1931, with 350 people on board.[75] By the end of 1933 the county had sponsored fifteen trains, carrying a total of 12,786 Mexicans.[76]

Because the campaign targeted relief recipients, it is likely that families visited by tuberculosis constituted a high proportion of the returnees. Antanacio Cordova entered the United States in 1912 and supported his wife and five children by working as an olive picker. Soon after he died from tuberculosis in 1922, the family applied for relief. They relied on such assistance off and on until 1932, when they returned to Mexico on a repatriation train.[77] We recall that the death of Emilia Castañeda De Valenciana's mother from tuberculosis devastated the family financially as well as emotionally. Because the father could find no employment as a stonemason or bricklayer, the mother had supported the household as a domestic worker. But after her death, the family lost their home and became dependent on county assistance. When asked how she got to Mexico, Emilia replied, "After my mother died, I guess my dad was pretty sad. Here he was left with a family, a couple of children to raise, no wife, no work and living off of welfare. . . . My dad asked the county to send him back to Mexico. . . . He knew he could get work there."[78]

Although Emilia emphasized her father's desire to return, other families impoverished by tuberculosis departed far less willingly. The administrative structure in Los Angeles facilitated the expansion of the notion of "public charge" to include the use of medical care. As already noted, the Department of Charities, the agency directing the repatriation drive, was responsible not just for the Bureau of Indigent Relief but also for Los Angeles General Hospital and Olive View Sanatorium; after 1932, its jurisdiction expanded to include most outpatient care delivered by the county. And department officials justified repatriation by pointing not just to the relief directed to Mexicans but also to the high cost of the health care services they received. On January 29, 1934, Rex Thomson, the superintendent of the department, wrote to Alejandro V. Martinez, the Mexican consul in Los Angeles, requesting his support for the repatriation campaign. "You will readily perceive," Thomson noted, that "the savings to the taxpayers due to the success of this repatriation has been tremendous." Those savings included not only the cost of the relief that would have been spent on the repatriates but also "the immense outstanding costs in the way of hospitalization, clinical and medical attention, and education facilities which this community is obligated to provide."[79] Thomson used virtually the same wording in a letter to the Los Angeles County Board of Supervisors on February 14, asking for more funds for Mexican repatriation.[80] Thirteen months later, he urged the board to endorse a resettlement plan in Mexico to encourage more immigrants to return, "thereby ultimately producing a tremendous savings, not only in the cost of relief . . . but also reducing materially the costs of relief afforded in our institutions to such indigent aliens and effecting a savings in the costs of other Governmental services afforded to them such as general health, educational, etc."[81]

No accounts survive of conversations between Department of Charities staff and individual Mexican clients. Two cases that came to the attention of the Board of Supervisors, however, demonstrate the determination of staff to rid the county of clients with large medical expenses. In both, the department requested funds to return the families to Mexico by car rather than on the organized train trips. The first, occurring in August 1930, involved a woman and her six children. According to the letter from a department social worker, the family received $67.50 in county aid each month. In addition, "The children present numerous health problems which require costly medical care." Federal immigration authorities had refused the department's request to deport the family but promised that if the family "can be taken to TiaJuana the immigration officer will prevent their return."[82] The second case, three years later, involved a couple with six children. The Superintendent of the Bureau of Welfare wrote that "the man and woman are both ill and represent an expensive case."[83]

To some extent, the repatriation drive represented a continuation of the policy of expulsion inaugurated by the Department of Charities in 1909. The pace of removals accelerated during the 1930s, when destitute migrants from other states poured into Los Angeles. But there were critical differences between the two programs. County officials pressured interstate migrants to return home only before they established residence. Mexicans, however, were repatriated regardless of the length of their residence in the county or state. The repatriation program thus clearly demonstrated that Mexicans could never consider Los Angeles home.

Moreover, by the 1930s, the Department of Charities had established a policy of returning sick interstate migrants only if they could find medical care at home. Although the department occasionally transported people in the absence of guarantees,[84] staff contacted local authorities and pressured them to promise to provide care. But the department was well aware that no medical assistance awaited the vast of majority of Mexican repatriates. In June 1934, Edythe Tate-Thompson referred to "the great numbers of tuberculous repatriates that were being left in various Mexican States without provision for care."[85] (Although that comment may have reflected an unusual display of solicitude for Mexicans, Tate-Thompson simply may have feared that many repatriates would again cross the border and thus pose a renewed threat to white Americans.)

The repatriation program also must have affected the health status of those left behind. Indeed, the program devastated Mexican communities in Los Angeles.[86] In an evaluation of the Huntington Park Mexican Colony, Violet Blanche Goldberg discussed the case of a woman who returned home two months after entering Olive View Sanatorium. In her absence, Goldberg wrote, "the cousin's family, also living in the house, had been repatriated through the efforts of the Department of Charities, and the home conditions were much improved."[87] But if the relatives' departure reduced overcrowding, it also may have removed the sources of care on which the woman depended. The loss of neighbors and friends often undoubtedly destroyed the social networks that are essential to healing.

On May 25, 1937, Rex Thomson wrote to the Board of Supervisors, requesting permission to hire five to ten social workers who "possess the ability to speak Spanish of extreme fluency" and could encourage indigent Mexicans to accept repatriation regardless of whether they were "employable or nonemployable."[88] By that date, indigent people deemed "employable" had been transferred to the rolls of the State Relief Administration or the federal Works Progress Administration. The County Department of Charities thus provided relief primarily to "unemployable" people, most of whom were sick or disabled. That department did, however, remain responsible for providing health care to all indigents, regardless of the source of their financial assistance.[89] The bulk of Thomson's letter consisted of an account of the "material and medical relief" furnished by the county. For the first time since the 1925 *Statistical Study*, specific figures were attached to the medical expenses associated with Mexicans.[90] The county spent $46,058 a month on material relief to "Mexican aliens" and another 74 percent as much for medical care ($30,395 for institutional care and $3,630 for outpatient care).[91]

Thomson attempted to reduce that burden in two ways. The Department of Charities transported four infirm people to Mexico in February 1938, two in May, four in August, and seven in October.[92] One historian writes that the repatriation program had "declined to the point where repatriates for the most part were . . . blind, tubercular, paralyzed, or were minor children or the aged."[93] The numbers involved certainly paled in comparison with those in earlier years, when trainloads of repatriates departed from Los Angeles. But these final trips also highlight a concern with the high cost of health care that had animated the program since its inception.

Tuberculosis was the diagnosis of approximately half the passengers on the 1938 trips.[94] That disease also was central to Thomson's second effort to reduce the cost of caring for Mexicans. At his behest, Gordon L. McDonough, a member of the Los Angeles County Board of Supervisors, traveled to Mexico in October 1938 to attempt to convince government officials to accept the return of Mexicans with tuberculosis. One problem was the paucity of available care. McDonough discovered that "the only tubercular hospital in Mexico is located at Talalpam, Huipulco. Dr. Donato Alarcon is director and the capacity is 180 beds."[95] But McDonough added that access was not the concern of Los Angeles County: "The question of whether this institution is inadequate or not is one for the Mexican government to determine."[96] That statement represented a radical departure from the policy vis-à-vis interstate migrants.

A much thornier issue revolved around the timing and place of infection. Describing his conversation with Ignacio Garcia Tellez, the Mexican secretary of the interior, McDonough wrote, "Concerning the tubercular cases, the question . . . arose as to whether these people had contracted tuberculosis in the United States or whether they were permitted to enter the United States with tuberculosis, after having passed the United States Health Service Examination."[97] McDonough claimed to find some support for his assertion that Mexicans imported tuberculosis in an interview with Dr. Walter Garnett, the U.S. Public Health Service official at El Paso responsible for administering medical examinations to people seeking visas for stays longer than 180 days. According to McDonough, Garnett stated that he "was allowed only $100.00 a month by the United States Government which did not provide sufficient funds for a detailed examination of people who may be afflicted with tubercular, venereal diseases or other contagious diseases."[98] Mexicans seeking permission to enter for shorter periods rarely received medical inspection.[99] The laxity of border control, of course, did not prove either that Mexico had high levels of tuberculosis or that many Mexicans suffered from the disease when they entered the United States. Indeed, McDonough's arguments failed to convince the Mexican government, which insisted that its nationals contracted TB in the United States.[100]

Shortly after receiving McDonough's report, the Los Angeles County Board of Supervisors directed J. H. O'Connor, the county counsel, to determine whether responsibility for the care of "Mexican aliens" with tuberculosis rested with Mexico or Los Angeles.[101] The issue rapidly became moot, however, in the face of the continued refusal of the Mexican government to accept the argument that it had an obligation to render such care.[102] On December 6, the Board of Supervisors rescinded its order to O'Connor.[103] Soon afterwards, all efforts to continue the repatriation program ended.

As a result of both deportation and repatriation, the Mexican population of Los Angeles declined by a third.[104] In 1932, the State Board of Health wrote, "The exodus of thousands of Mexicans from this State has reduced both our clinic and hospital population with reference to this group."[105] The silence about the effect of these campaigns on the health status of Mexicans both in Los Angeles and at home was striking.

The 1930s saw not only a massive onslaught against Mexicans throughout the Southwest but also some of their first significant community activism. A major organization was El Congreso de Pueblos que Hablan Español (the National Congress of Spanish Speaking Peoples), which was especially prominent in Los Angeles.[106] Although the group was associated primarily with labor struggles and political protest, a recent study demonstrates that it also focused on health.[107] A few months before the inaugural convention in Los Angeles in April 1939, leaders sent a petition to the L.A. City Council asking for the "promotion and extension of government subsidized health projects, and slum clearance projects, to protect the health of the people."[108] Like Pomeroy, El Congreso blamed the government officials responsible for the dismal housing conditions in Mexican areas. But Pomeroy also implicated the poor housekeeping of Mexican women, the large size of their families, and the special vulnerability of Mexican bodies to the disease. The petition made no mention of cultural or physical differences. The council committee to which the petition was referred filed it away and then promptly ignored it. Nevertheless, the group continued to focus on health issues, demanding improved housing and access to care.[109]

El Congreso also challenged state and local health officials by insisting that Mexican workers were entitled to an equal share of social benefits. Although the group encouraged all Mexicans to become citizens, it also argued that noncitizens should be accorded the same rights. One leader articulated the organization's position: "These people are not aliens—they have contributed their endurance, sacrifices, youth and labor to the Southwest. Indirectly, they have paid more taxes than all the stockholders of California's industrialized agriculture, the sugar beet companies and the large cotton interests that operate or have operated with the labor of Mexican workers."[110] That statement directly challenged Tate-Thompson as well as Pomeroy. While those officials repeatedly described Mexicans as liabilities because they paid no taxes but required expensive medical care, El Congreso stressed that the state's economic well-being rested on Mexican labor.

After noting the decline of Mexican patients in both clinics and hospitals, the California State Board of Health wrote in 1932: "Filipinos constitute one of our worst problems at the present time. Many of them are food handlers, either working in fields with fresh fruits or vegetables or working in kitchens and restaurants."[111] Because the Philippines was a U.S. territory, the large numbers of Filipinos who arrived in California in the late 1920s were considered "nationals."

By the early 1930s, Los Angeles had become an important center for that population. As the Board of Health noted, many found employment in service work as well as in agriculture; a very high proportion were young, single men.[112]

Pressure to expel Filipinos arose in the 1920s and intensified after the advent of the depression. As in the campaign for Mexican repatriation, an important charge was that members of the population created social problems by importing "loathsome diseases" and requiring expensive medical care.[113] The nativists' first significant victory was the 1934 passage of the Tydings McDuffie Act, establishing the Philippines as a commonwealth and changing the status of Filipinos from nationals to aliens.[114] The 1935 Repatriation Act, introduced by California congressman Robert Welch, provided for the return of "Filipino wards of public and private organizations" as well as others who were unemployed.[115] Although Welch originally had proposed that the war and navy departments furnish military transports, the government contracted with private steamship companies.[116] Very few Filipinos, however, accepted the offer of free transportation home.[117]

Health officials helped to fuel the nativist campaign. Edythe Tate-Thompson's monthly reports document her relentless hostility toward Filipinos and her tireless efforts in support of expulsion. After visiting Kern General Hospital in April 1933, she complained:

> Here, as in many of the other general hospitals, the beds on the tuberculosis service were nearly all filled with Filipinos. These people seem to have more complications than other races. Rarely do I see a Filipino with just a pulmonary involvement. They require very much more nursing than a white patient, and since they are so often disturbed mentally, coupled with certain groups of them carrying many superstitions, it makes life very miserable for white patients around them.[118]

Tate-Thompson also insisted that, like Mexicans, Filipinos and other Asians did not deserve high-quality care. "Naturally I do not expect San Joaquin County, with a ward filled with Orientals to maintain a standard such as they have at their sanatorium in the mountains," she wrote in June 1934.[119]

In addition, Tate-Thompson joined the campaign for removal. At the suggestion of John Porter, the president of the California State Board of Health, she conferred in February 1933 with the Federal Immigration Officer in Los Angeles, who suggested that she cooperate "in urging the new Congress to pass the bill returning Filipinos on army transports."[120] At a meeting of the State Board of Health two months later, she requested permission to raise the issue of the "deportation of aliens" with the California Conference of Social Agencies.[121] The resolution she submitted in May began by noting that more than 30,000

Filipinos lived in California and that tuberculosis was the cause of a third of the deaths. In an explicit reference to the "likely to become a public charge" clause of the immigration statute, the resolution argued that the high prevalence of tuberculosis "constitutes dependency as these people must occupy beds in county hospitals and be cared for at public expense." The resolution concluded by recommending that California congressmen seek passage of the repatriation bill "and that it be stipulated that Army transports be used to return these unfortunate dependent people to their own country at the earliest possible moment."[122] The conference's refusal to vote on the resolution prompted Tate-Thompson to remark that social workers "seldom see the complications in the present social disorder."[123]

On a trip to Washington, D.C., in August, Tate-Thompson met with the commissioner of immigration to urge him to work for "voluntary deportation" of Filipinos. As she later wrote, "I mentioned to him the great amount of sickness, particularly tuberculosis, among them at the present time; and the fact that they were filling up our hospital beds for almost indefinite periods; and I thought perhaps a recommendation from him to the War Department might make it possible to use these transports without legislation."[124] Again, she met opposition. According to her report, the commissioner responded that California "had a distinct obligation to take care of any sick Filipino, regardless of what their illness might be, or the length of time they had been in the state." His second objection was "that very little had been done in the Philippine Islands, either to provide care, or diagnosis for the Filipinos, so that if they were returned on army transports, we would merely be creating a difficult position in the Philippine Islands." But that argument too failed to convince Tate-Thompson: "I was quite interested to see how indifferent they were as to the problems here," she concluded.[125]

Local as well as state officials sought Filipino repatriation. In April 1934 the *Los Angeles Herald* reported that Frank L. Shaw, chairman of the Los Angeles County Board of Supervisors, planned to inaugurate a program to return Filipinos on the relief rolls and that Supervisor Roger W. Jessup asked the county counsel to determine the program's legality.[126] Despite the passage of the federal Repatriation Act the following year, the Department of Charities proceeded on its own, contracting with American steamship companies to transport indigents to Manila at reduced rates.[127] As in the case of Mexican repatriation, sick and disabled people were especially likely to be encouraged to depart. An M.A. social work thesis included this account: "It was the privilege of the writer to work with some of the Filipinos who were on relief at the Los Angeles County Welfare office in the spring of 1936. Most of these people were sickly and unable to work. Because of their inability to work, it was often suggested that it was perhaps best for them to be sent back to their families and immediate relatives in the homeland. They were told that they would receive better care at home."[128] Only a few Filipinos agreed to leave.

Filipino immigrants with tuberculosis appear in a very different light in Carlos Bulosan's semifictional autobiography. Published in 1946, *America Is in the Heart* rapidly achieved the status of a classic.[129] Bulosan's friend P. C. Morantte, a Filipino journalist, concluded that the book is "30% autobiography, 40% case history of Pinoy [Filipino immigrant] life in America, and 30% fiction."[130] Like other commentators, I refer to the narrator as Carlos to distinguish him from the historical Bulson.[131]

Born into an impoverished farm family in the Philippines, Carlos worked rather than attending school as a child. He broke both an arm and a leg falling from a tree and almost drowned in a river. Other tragedies struck his family. A younger sister died, one brother narrowly avoided a forced marriage, and another was viciously beaten. When his parents lost their small plot of land, they faced desperate poverty.

Arriving in depression-era Seattle, Carlos traveled up and down the West Coast, finding work in canneries and the fields and occasionally as a dishwasher and houseboy. He was beaten in a box car while trying to protect a woman from rape and again in San Diego "by restaurant and hotel proprietors."[132] Other men lost limbs in accidents and were hurt in brawls; a few were murdered. Worst of all was his sense of degradation. He began to steal, cheat at cards, and carry a gun and knife. What saved him was his conversion to socialism and participation in the labor movement. Simultaneously, he realized he had a mission as a writer. When his poems won a friend's praise, he "knew surely" he "had become a new man." He "could fight the world now" with his "mind," not merely his "hands."[133]

But illness suddenly derailed him. He was living with his brother Macario in Los Angeles when he started "to cough" and "could not sleep at night." While reading new poems aloud, he "began to cough violently and could not stop." Soon he found himself "coughing out blood." When Macario arrived home, he called a doctor. " 'I'm afraid it is TB,' he said. 'Advanced stage. I'm sorry.' "[134]

While most narratives of people with tuberculosis during the 1920s and 1930s "offer a lengthy, defensive, apologetic explanation" of how and why they contracted the disease,[135] Carlos stated simply, "The years of hunger had caught up with me."[136] By viewing social injustice as the cause of his illness, he avoided some of the stigma surrounding it. Unlike the predominantly white, middle-class patients who wrote about their experiences, Carlos had seen too many wounded bodies to expect to be able to avoid serious illness and injury. He also was not the first family member to suffer from the disease. After returning from war, Carlos's older brother Luciano had grown "thinner," coughed at night," and had "a sad shine in his eyes"; he died several years later of tuberculosis.[137]

Macario thus immediately understood the meaning of Carlos's diagnosis. He would "have to wait for slow death." Carlos, however, commented, "At first I did not realize the extent of the disease. I did not know that it would incapacitate me for years. But during the first days of anxiety, lying in bed alone and thinking of my interrupted work, I had only one desire: to get well as soon as possible and go back to the labor movement."[138] His diagnosis disrupted Macario's life as well as his own. Because he was the most intellectually gifted of the brothers, the parents had sent him to school and invested considerable hope in his ultimate success. Although he had held menial jobs in America, he too found a sense of purpose in socialism. Instead of joining the workers' struggle, however, he was forced to find a job making salads and pastries in an Italian restaurant to support Carlos.

We do not learn who made the decision that Carlos should enter the hospital, how long he had to wait for a bed, or how he finally gained admittance. He tells us only that in June "an ambulance came to take me to the Los Angeles County Hospital." This was not his first experience of American medical care. He and a friend were climbing aboard a freight train when a railroad detective attacked them. Although Carlos fled, his friend was seriously hurt. At the hospital, "a kind doctor and two nurses assured us that they would do their best for him.[139] Carlos could only "wonder at the paradox of America." His comrade had been beaten, "and yet in this hospital, among white people . . . we had found refuge and tolerance."[140] But now Carlos was the patient and his stay would last months, not days. Like many people with TB, he initially viewed placement as confinement. On the ride he "watched the buildings, committing them to memory" because he knew he "would not see them for a long time"; he soon realized that his ward was "above the hospital jail."[141]

In one major way, however, his response differed dramatically from that of other residents of long-term care institutions. According to one anthropologist, visitors "often find that the patients are rather indifferent to news of the outside world, preferring instead to talk about other patients in the room, their doctors, and the events of the floor."[142] Several patients did profoundly affect Carlos. He enjoyed his time with "Panagros, the Greek" and "Sobel, the Jew."[143] Penning a letter for an illiterate boy from Arkansas, Carlos felt as if he were "writing to all the unhappy mothers whose sons left and did not return."[144] The courage of a ten-year-old whose arms had been amputated made Carlos feel "at once brave and ashamed."[145] On the eve of his departure, he recalled the "genuine friends, who had sat with me in the hopeless hours, the black days of my operations."[146]

Nevertheless, he remained focused on the visitors who kept him in touch with struggles at home and abroad. They, too, provided heroic models. Some, for example, came to say good-bye before leaving to confront death in the Spanish Civil War. About one, Carlos commented that he "gave meaning to the futilities of other men's lives."[147] Others brought the books which enabled Carlos to use his hospital stay to fulfill his dream of education. Immersing himself in works by such diverse writers as Hart Crane, Jack London, Mikhail Sholokhov, Federico Garcia Lorca, Alexander Pushkin, and André Malraux, Carlos became "a lost man in the hospital." Unable to "converse with the other patients because of their intellectual sterility,"[148] he found "spiritual kinship" with the authors he read.[149] Between visits, he sent frequent letters, thus maintaining contact with friends and comrades while honing his skills as a writer.

Suffering added a sense of urgency to Carlos's studies. An old knee injury caused "shooting pain," and he endured three operations, including the removal of the ribs on his right side. A doctor told him he would live "for a while." Death surrounded him. His ward was "overflowing with dying men."[150] When his condition deteriorated, he was transferred to a small room where three other men were "waiting to die"; at the end, they lay "gasping for the last bit of air."[151] He read "ceaselessly, suffering, trying to forget that I was dying."[152] While "other patients were worrying and complaining," he was able to bore "through the earth's core, leveling all seas and oceans, swimming in the constellations."[153] When he received a letter informing him that his brother Luciano had died of tuberculosis, Carlos "crept out of the bed and cried in the bathroom, holding my chest for fear the blood would burst out of my own perforated lungs." Standing in the darkness, he

> remembered all my years in the Philippines, my father fighting for his inherited land, my mother selling *boggong* to the impoverished peasants. I remembered all my brothers and their bitter fight for a place in the sun, their tragic fear that they might not live long enough to contribute something vital to the world. I remembered my own swift and dangerous life in America. And I cried, recalling all the years that had come and gone, but my remembrance gave me a strange courage and the vision of a better life.
>
> "Yes, I will be a writer and make all of you live again my worlds," I sobbed.[154]

But the literature he devoured could not hide the wretched conditions of the hospital or protect him from discrimination. Awakening after surgery, he saw a "clean, well-lighted room. . . . Everything smelled fresh and new; evidently I was in the new building."[155] Soon, however, he returned to his "dark" and "dismal ward."[156] After two years, he applied "to be transferred to a sanitarium for complete recovery," only to discover that the Social Service Department used "technical reasons" to eliminate "certain patients from relief care."[157] Because he had arrived in the United States as a minor, he needed a guardian to sign certain papers; lacking one, he was deemed ineligible to enter a sanatorium. Carlos "began to feel like the Mexicans who thought the doctors were killing them off because there were too many of them."[158] When he appealed his rejection, a social worker "came, not to help me but to tell me there was racism even in the Los Angeles County Hospital. 'You Filipinos,' she said calmly, 'ought to be shipped back to your jungle homes.' "[159]

Unsuccessful in his attempt, Carlos decided to depart. It was not an easy choice: "I was afraid to leave the hospital. I knew that a perilous life awaited me outside. . . . I had never known peace, except in the hospital, where there was always something to eat, and a place to sleep on the cold nights."[160] Nevertheless, he now had "an unswerving intellectual weapon" to use. "Maybe I would win this time, and if I did—would I not create a legend of courage and valor that other poor young men could emulate?"

It is possible to substantiate some parts of this story. The historical record demonstrates that Bulosan contracted tuberculosis, enrolled in L.A. County Hospital, underwent lung surgery, experienced serious knee pain, and read voraciously.[161] P. C. Morantte recalled visiting Bulosan in the hospital after an operation and seeing "in his beardless face, his pale sunken cheeks, not the pallor of looming death but the incandescent light of hope glinting in his eyes, a latent energy coming to the surface from a deep source of life."[162] After the completion of the new hospital building, Edythe Tate-Thompson insisted that tuberculosis patients remain in the old facility, lest they find the surroundings so attractive they try to extend their stays. The ward to which Carlos returned after surgery was thus probably as miserable as he stated. And some aspects of Bulosan's account which cannot be verified nevertheless ring true. It is not far-fetched to assume that, during the repatriation campaigns, many Mexicans felt unsafe in public hospitals and that Filipino patients who asked to transfer to Olive View were urged to return home instead.

Nevertheless, the significance of the book lies not in the accuracy of its details but rather in the contrast if offers to official texts. Ignoring the perspectives of Mexicans and Filipinos with tuberculosis, health authorities stressed the resources they consumed and the germs they potentially spread. Because Bulosan remained in the county hospital for two years and was the brother of a restaurant worker, he was especially likely to have been depicted as both a burden and a menace. Instead, he defined himself as a uniquely valuable individual and told a story of growing personal dignity and power.

Chapter 7

"Agitation over the Migrant Issue"

Rafael Garcia must have been desperate by the time he applied for help from a Los Angeles office of the State Relief Administration (SRA) on November 20, 1936.[1] Two of his five children, sixteen-year-old Enrique and thirteen-year-old Maria, were in the tuberculosis ward of Los Angeles General Hospital. His wife, Gloria, was pregnant. And the money he had earned picking fruit during the summer was completely gone.[2]

But the SRA had little to offer. According to the case file, Rafael's legal residence was Globe, Arizona, where he had worked as recently as June, and the staff thus made plans for the family's "immediate transportation." Unable to challenge the decision directly, Rafael raised two objections. The first was that he had a 1929 Ford coupe, which he wanted to drive back to Globe. When the SRA decided that it would be cheaper to send all the family members by train rather than pay for some to travel by car, he "refused to sell the car and return with his family on the train." His second objection was that his wife was too close to delivery to be able to travel. The SRA thus referred Gloria to a doctor, who certified that the due date was still four months away and she therefore could safely depart. When Rafael still refused to sell his car, he was informed that "if he refused to return by train, his family was to be sent back without him and he would have to get back through his own efforts."[3]

Meanwhile, two-year-old Ernesto was "taken seriously ill." The SRA sent a physician who "personally took the child to the General Hospital," and he too was diagnosed with tuberculosis. Now the agency had an added incentive to expel the entire family as quickly as possible. But new difficulties arose. The Southern Pacific Railroad had sleeping cars only for the trip to Bowie, Arizona.

The hospital social worker decided that Maria and Ernesto could sit in the day coach during the five-hour trip from Bowie to Globe, but that "some arrangements would have to be made for Enrique to lie down during the entire trip as the child was hemorrhaging continuously, and he was urgently in need of pneumothorax treatments which had not been started pending his return to his legal residence." After "several wires had been sent," the railroad agreed to allow Enrique to travel in the baggage car from Bowie to Globe.[4]

Then, on the day before the family was due to leave, the hospital doctors decided that the younger children, too, needed bed rest throughout the trip. The Southern Pacific baggage agent first promised to provide three cots and bed clothing but rescinded that offer the following day. "This information was given to the medical worker at the General Hospital who advised that the hospital had no way of providing these things and that it was so imperative that the three children be gotten out of the hospital that, if necessary, in spite of the doctors' orders, they would have to sit up in the day coach during the last five hours of the trip." Because the SRA supervisors refused to "be a party to transportation unless satisfactory arrangements could be made for the three children," the hospital finally agreed to supply "three cots, three mattresses and ample bedding."[5]

Ten minutes before the scheduled departure time, the ambulances still had not arrived at the station. A phone call to the medical social worker disclosed that the superintendent of the Globe public hospital had just announced that he could not accept the children without proof of the family's legal residence. When he finally received verification, he consented to their return. Gloria and her children left for Globe on February 11, 1937. Both the General Hospital and the SRA "sent wires advising the time of arrival and requesting that ambulances meet the family at the train as they were in need of immediate hospitalization." Rafael returned later by car.[6]

The Garcia family were part of a vast cohort of migrants who poured into California during the 1930s, alarming health and welfare officers, igniting intense political conflicts, and engendering a new round of exclusionary policies. The state contained just 4.7 percent of the population of the nation as a whole but 13.5 percent of the recipients of aid from the Federal Transient Service between 1933 and 1935.[7] Los Angeles grew especially rapidly. By 1940, its population had increased 26 percent, compared to 21 percent for the state as a whole.[8] Not surprisingly, then, the metropolis quickly became a center of the antimigrant campaign.

It is highly likely that Rafael Garcia's country of origin contributed to the harsh treatment he received. With three tubercular children in Los Angeles

General Hospital, the Garcias epitomized the burdensome Mexican family county officials were determined to expel.[9] But if the hostility directed against Mexicans was unusually vehement, they were not the only group to encounter contempt and discrimination. Poor whites arriving between 1935 and 1937 from the "dust bowl" states (Oklahoma, Texas, Arkansas, and Missouri) also received extremely negative attention.[10]

When answering investigators, migrants from all parts of the country cited better jobs as their primary reason for moving. According to a 1929 report, however, ill health was "second to employment as a displacing factor."[11] A higher proportion of migrants from Arizona (the home state of the Garcia family) than of those from the nation as a whole sought improved health (one-fifth, as opposed to one-tenth of migrants in general).[12] Gloria Garcia had brought her children to Los Angeles because she was not "satisfied with medical care" in Globe and wanted them in "a good hospital."[13] Other health seekers still believed in the healing power of California sunshine. Despite all the attempts by public health authorities to convince East Coast people suffering from tuberculosis to stay home, some doctors continued to advise them to avoid snow and ice. And now dust storms in the drought-ridden states added to the environmental hazards tuberculosis sufferers were urged to flee.[14]

In many cases, there was no single cause of migration. A California investigator concluded in 1934, "Back in the minds of many transients who come to California to get work there also lies the thought of health."[15] One man's story demonstrates how a desire for better health could intermingle with other incentives. A Russian immigrant, David Lubin was a garment worker in New York in 1938 when he found a newspaper ad placed by two young women who wanted to share the expenses of a car trip to Los Angeles. Interviewed in 2002, he remembered what "an adventure" it was "to come across the country." And Los Angeles "was a whole different world," with "orange groves, tangerines, and lemons." He also had family ties there. Because his parents had died when he was young, his two sisters had always been especially important to him. One had moved to Los Angeles with her husband and now had a boy. When the sister was diagnosed with tuberculosis soon after the husband deserted, David decided to move close to his nephew. Because Los Angeles was another center of the garment industry, David assumed he would be able to find employment. And he had pressing physical concerns himself. After contracting tuberculosis several years earlier, he had spent time in a sanatorium in Liberty, New York. Although he had recovered, eastern winters seemed particularly "gruesome," and many people advised him that permanent cure was possible only in Southern California.[16]

Regardless of the impetus for the trip, serious health problems plagued the migrant population. A 1936 San Diego study found that "diet changes caused by lack of sufficient funds . . . often resulted in the occurrence of rickets, pellagra, scurvy, secondary anemia and other causes of malnutrition, which tend to make the patient susceptible to more serious diseases such as tuberculosis."[17] Dr. William P. Shepard, the president of the Western Branch of the American Public Health Association, concluded in 1940 that "migrants as a whole are far from a healthy group" and that tuberculosis was common, "especially among young adults."[18]

Many sick migrants hesitated to apply for health care, fearing that once they attracted official notice, they would be sent home—a reasonable concern throughout the 1930s.[19] Those who sought medical care found little available. The Garcia family received out-patient care from both a doctor who confirmed that Gloria could travel and another who "personally" took Ernesto to the hospital. Both physicians were part of the SRA health-care program. Doctors who agreed to serve on local medical panels were assigned cases on a rotating basis. But federal regulations stipulated that the doctors could furnish only acute care, not the long-term services people with tuberculosis needed. And because eligibility was restricted to SRA clients, most people failed to qualify.[20]

Migrants with tuberculosis thus remained dependent on the overcrowded county and city outpatient clinics. A key argument that health director John L. Pomeroy gave for refusing to transfer TB diagnosis and care to the County Department of Charities was that the Health Department was not subject to the state residence law and thus could serve all indigent people, regardless of the length of time they had lived in the county or state. In 1934, he estimated that nonresidents represented 40 percent of the clientele of his tuberculosis clinics.[21]

The state residence law did, however, apply to the two institutions operated by the County Department of Charities. As a result, Olive View Sanatorium was completely closed to nonresidents after 1931. The county hospital continued to accept new arrivals, but only if they were "in dire distress"; people with TB had to be hemorrhaging in order to qualify.[22] The case files of various relief agencies suggest that the facility routinely rejected patients with "far advanced" disease.[23] In 1937, Pomeroy complained that his department often found "cases of tuberculosis within a migratory family," but could not "arrange satisfactory institutional medical care." As he pointed out, new therapies had made hospital placement especially urgent: "Treatment of tuberculosis has changed so radically during the past few years, and surgery is so often used now-a-days that it seems quite unfortunate that early cases of tuberculosis, whether among residents or non-residents, cannot receive the benefits of modern medical science."[24] The

Garcia case indicates that the hospital delayed surgery for at least some tubercular nonresidents who did gain admission and then discharged them prematurely. Although sixteen-year-old Enrique was "hemorrhaging continuously" and thus "urgently in need of pneumothorax treatments," those had "not been started pending his return to his legal residence."

In 1940 Governor Culbert L. Olson wrote that California had "been torn by agitation over the migrant issue almost continuously from 1931 to date."[25] Health officials participated in that agitation in familiar ways. One was by alerting the public to the dangers the newcomers posed. Dr. Shepard, for example, invoked the common argument that "contagious diseases are no respecters of social class or geographic boundary." As a result, the health problems of "destitute migrants" were "serious, not only to the migrants themselves but to the communities in which they settle."[26] Ironically, the dearth of affordable health services exacerbated fears. In 1938 the Los Angeles Tuberculosis and Health Association reported that a "comprehensive survey of the transient population" had revealed that "there are not sufficient facilities to care for those who are ill and a menace to the established population."[27] Others reminded the public that migrants who spread disease also inflicted a financial toll. In 1936, Edythe Tate-Thompson, director of the Bureau of Tuberculosis, found cases in which "as many as eight migratory people in one family all [had] tuberculosis, with a record of the father and mother and five other children dying." As a result, "one has to wonder if one should not make a comparative cost of one case of human plague against those migratory groups, moving centers of infection wherever they go. Eventually they will acquire a residence and isolation will run into millions of dollars."[28]

Health officials also buttressed the campaign against migrants by claiming expertise not only about their physical status but also about their personal characteristics. George Parish, the director of the Los Angeles City Department of Health, described the typical migrant woman as "a drudge" and the children as a "happy-go-lucky lot" who "roam the streets." He explained high venereal disease rates this way: "In their "cramped quarters . . . toilet facilities are at the end of the hall, common property for all the families. Streams of half-clothed people are coming from or going to it. They become acquainted and familiarity causes them to become careless and indifferent. This familiarity causes a fertile field for gonorrhea and syphilis, to say nothing of other diseases."[29]

Eugenic beliefs dominated Edythe Tate-Thompson's writings. Having "seen quite a good deal of these people," she was "convinced that the majority of those coming from Oklahoma and Arkansas" were "primitives"; she doubted that "the older group" could be "educated into any modern methods."[30] Regardless of their place of origin, all migrants were, in Tate-Thompson's view, a shiftless group who took unfair advantage of public assistance programs.[31] In December 1938 she focused on a Texas family who arrived in California "several years ago," settled for a time in Imperial County, and now lived in Long Beach. The Bureau of Tuberculosis "has known the family over quite a period of years, and has given them as much advice and help as we could. The help they took; the advice they paid no attention to." The father and oldest son had been "confined in the tuberculosis hospital for six months" in Imperial County. Tate-Thompson's "impression at the time was that it was a very early tuberculosis and that they were hungry more than anything else." Although county authorities insisted the family return to Texas when the woman gave birth to her fifth child, they were soon back in California. "By this time the woman had learned nearly all of the ropes necessary, and she rather welcomed the fact that the father had tuberculosis, because she thought she was going to get some help on that basis for the children." Tate-Thompson then lost track of the family for a period, largely, she thought, because she would not help them "panhandle all over the state." Recently, however, "the woman came in the office, claiming that she had to have more help. The primary goal was to get the husband in a hospital so that she could get state aid for the children."[32]

Tate-Thompson also sought to shift financial responsibility for migrants from the state to the federal government. That effort could, of course, be construed as an attempt to obtain adequate resources for the population. But the tenor of Tate-Thompson's comments leaves little doubt that, as with her support of the 1916 Kent Bill, her major objective was to repel sick migrants, not care for them. In 1932 she stressed the financial burdens they imposed: "Federal legislation is necessary to collect from States for the indigent, delinquent and sick who cross the border of this State. Fruits and vegetables are inspected at the border, yet they cost little compared to the cost of education, delinquency and illness to a group who pay no taxes and are a liability on each community."[33] In 1936, she would complain about the consequences of ignoring her request: "If we had had four years ago when the opportunity presented itself the cooperation we needed, hundreds and hundreds of people who are far advanced cases of tuberculosis and who ultimately will have to be admitted to our hospitals as emergency cases could have been sent out of the state."[34]

Local officials joined the campaign to prevent the migration of people with tuberculosis. In a 1932 letter asking for authorization to send a delegate to the annual meeting of the National Tuberculosis Association, John L. Pomeroy, director of the County Department of Health, explained that "the subject is of enormous economic importance to Los Angeles County particularly because of the great burden that is thrust upon the county by persons who come here because of this disease." The previous year he had succeeded in "getting the National [Tuberculosis] Association to send a request to every public health authority in the United States to discourage persons coming to California this year for tuberculosis." Pomeroy believed that "request has resulted in a marked decline in the number of cases coming here this year." The proposed delegate for the forthcoming meeting would "do everything possible to interest the National Association to urge the various cities and states in this country that tuberculosis can be cured as well at home as it can in California."[35]

Because the Federal Transient Service provided material relief to migrants, its establishment in May 1933 temporarily muted the agitation. Nevertheless, Tate-Thompson continued to press for more vigorous action. Her monthly report for August 1933 read: "On the 17th I attended the meeting called by the Emergency Relief Administrator to discuss the problem of transients in the State. On the following morning I spoke on a plan that could be devised to stop migration."[36] In May 1934, she protested the "fact that up to the present time the Emergency Relief is side-stepping the problem of the transient tuberculous and his family."[37]

After the liquidation of the Transient Service in September 1935, the campaign against migrants revived with redoubled energy. The first and most dramatic response was the notorious "Bum Brigade," organized by Los Angeles police chief, James E. Davis. In early 1936 Davis sent 125 officers to the border to prevent indigents from entering the state. Although county organizations praised the blockade for attempting "to turn back these hordes of unwelcome invaders,"[38] it provoked outrage and ridicule throughout the nation. When the American Civil Liberties Union challenged the patrol in court, Davis finally conceded defeat.[39]

Davis later claimed that he had devised the plan in consultation with the sheriff's office, the railroads, and two groups with jurisdiction over many TB patients, the County Department of Charities and state relief agencies.[40] Tate-Thompson too appears to have given her endorsement. In autumn 1936, when Davis was considering reinstating the patrol, she reported, "Many interviews have taken place this past month with reference to the migratory laborer. The Chief of Police gave a luncheon to a great many people representing various organizations." The purpose was "to give Chief Davis support on this plan for Border Patrol. . . . There was discussion over a registration card with finger prints, but evidently this is not possible. Very lax methods exist at the border beyond the examination of cotton and fruit for boll weevil and fruit fly and a registration of the machines by the Motor Vehicle Department. The lame, the halt, and the blind come across without notice being given them. It is to laugh when one considers the cost of illness, illiteracy, and delinquency compared with the fruit fly and the boll weevil."[41]

Tate-Thompson's repeated references to the plant quarantine stations on the border suggests she also may have supported a legislative attempt to use them to examine migrants. The Redwine-Jones Bill, introduced by two Los Angeles assemblymen in 1935, sought to prevent the entry of "all paupers, vagabonds, indigent persons and persons likely to become public charges and all persons affected with contagious or infectious disease."[42] In 1939, an unsuccessful attempt was made to resurrect the bill "to preserve the public peace, health, and safety" of the state.[43]

The late 1930s also saw renewed attempts to shift responsibility for "transient relief" to the federal government. In April 1936, Pomeroy again requested funds to send a representative to a conference organized by the National Tuberculosis Association. This time "various federal, state, and local officials" would meet in Santa Fe "to consider the problem of tuberculosis among transients." That, he noted, "is a difficult problem in which Los Angeles County is tremendously interested."[44] A few months later, he reported that the meeting had "resulted in a set of recommendations satisfactory to both medical and social work groups, and a set of resolutions endorsing Federal Grants-in-Aid to States for the care of the transient tuberculous, with an emphasis on the need of referring this problem to the United States Public Health Service."[45]

Not all "medical groups," however, were equally pleased with the outcome. Describing the meeting in her monthly report, Tate-Thompson noted she was "surprised to find how little the Health Officers knew about the migratory transient laborer with reference to tuberculosis and how few of the State Tuberculosis Secretaries had any knowledge of the fact that there was a problem." It was thus "small wonder" that she and the Arizona representatives soon realized "that we were not put on the planning committee for the simple reason that anything we might have suggested would be too practical and might hasten the day." Furthermore, because "legal obstacles" would prevent the Public Health Service from assuming responsibility for the migrant population, the resolutions adopted at the meeting would "amount to very little." If California continued to depend "on the National Tuberculosis Association with their headquarters in New York," the result would be that "things [would] drag along indefinitely without any action."[46] Nevertheless, there was some cause for optimism: "The friends in Arizona who speak my language and who know we can do something have written me that they feel California and Arizona should join hands." Tate-Thompson hoped to be able to present "practical" suggestions to the State Board of Health, involving demands on the federal government "to provide either an abandoned Army post or in wards of the Veterans' Bureau hospitals care for the people with tuberculosis." In conclusion, she reminded the board that "this state is going to pay the price, running into millions of dollars in the next three years, for what we require with these thousands of people who have crossed the border, many of them ill and who must be hospitalized."[47]

In July 1937, Tate-Thompson reported she was "working with the Supervisors, particularly in Los Angeles, to see how much pressure can be brought to bear on Harry Hopkins for care of the [migrant] sick."[48] (One of President Roosevelt's chief advisers, Hopkins held top administrative positions in the Federal Emergency Relief Administration, the Civil Works Administra-tion, and the Works Progress Administration.) Pomeroy's report for 1936–37 stated that he had "appealed to the Federal and State Government" in "relation to the problem of the transient."[49] The following year he wrote that he had spent "considerable time" in "gaining support for the principle that the Federal Government should assume financial responsibility for the care of needy nonresidents, including the sick."[50]

Once again, exclusion shaded easily into expulsion. Relief offices throughout the United States historically had used the settlement laws to transport nonresident applicants back to their communities of origin. The pace of removals quickened throughout the United States during the 1930s.[51] The two California agencies responsible for returning indigent migrants were the State Relief Administration and the County Department of Charities. As an "able-bodied" unemployed man, Rafael Garcia had come under the purview of the SRA. Eleven months before he made his application, that agency had instituted a policy of discontinuing assistance to clients who refused to return to their legal residences. In 1938, the rules became even more restrictive; now nonresidents could receive assistance only if they promised in advance to return to their home communities.[52] During the five years ending in 1940, the California SRA sent 25,213 back to their legal residence.[53] In Los Angeles, more than 2,800 departed in 1938 alone.[54]

Because the Department of Charities had jurisdiction over "unemployable" indigents, its clientele included many sick and disabled people. Its residence requirements, however, were even more rigid than those of the SRA. Applicants who had not lived in the state for three years and the county for one were eligible only for "emergency" assistance, typically lasting three days.[55] Then they were offered tickets out. During 1937 and 1938, the department transported approximately ninety clients a month (as opposed to less than four a month in 1913).[56]

The paucity of surviving documents makes it impossible to calculate the proportion of tuberculosis sufferers in that large, forced, reverse migration. Nevertheless, some evidence indicates that families likes the Garcias, with many afflicted members, represented a disproportionate share of the returnees, just as they had of Mexican and Filipino repatriates. As Tate- Thompson remarked in February 1936, "every effort" was made to get nonresident tuberculosis patients "out of the state at the earliest possible moment."[57] Rex Thomson, the director of the County Department of Charities, used the same argument for transporting tubercular migrants that he had employed to justify the removal of seriously ill Mexicans. The files of the Board of Supervisors contain several letters written by either him or A. C. Price, the superintendent of the Bureau of County Welfare, asking for funds to provide special accommodations (usually a separate compartment on the train and the services of an attendant) for tubercular clients who agreed to depart. In each case, Thomson or Price explained that the cost of continuing to provide long-term care for the patient would far exceed the one-time expense of those accommodations—a particularly crucial consideration after the onset of the depression.[58]

Health authorities supported the drive to expel migrants in various ways. Tate-Thompson often pressed both the SRA and the County Department of Charities to transport sick clients and helped to arrange the trips.[59] Medical social workers played similar roles. The social worker at the Los Angeles General Hospital believed it was "so imperative" to remove the Garcia children that she had insisted that they could travel in the coach section of the train, "in spite of the doctors' orders." Zudenka Buben, the chief of the Division of Medical Society Service in the County Department of Health, discussed the case of a "non-resident American orphan boy, aged 16 years" who attended the Compton tuberculosis clinic in 1933. Because he was "mentally delinquent" and a "food handler" and lived with a married sister who had a small child, he was considered a menace as well as a financial drain. The clinic physician "recommended hospital care, but since [the boy] was a non-resident, he was ineligible for any of the county institutions, and there were no financial resources within the family to permit private institutional care." The best solution was thus expulsion. "This boy would have continued to run the streets, and have become a burden on Los Angeles County had it not been for the quick action of the County Health Department diagnosing the case, giving him close supervision and helping arrange the plan to have him returned to his legal residence."[60]

Nevertheless, it was far easier to arrange the trips than to make them happen. Both the SRA and Department of Charities were required to obtain authorization from local officials in the migrants' place of origin. But many had lost legal residence.[61] In addition, virtually all had come from parts of the country deeply hurt by the depression. As a result, the local officials to whom the SRA and Department of Charities appealed tended to be overwhelmed with their own growing case loads and reluctant to add to them. The county received permission to send a "separated white man, 27 years of age" with "pulmonary tuberculosis" to a hospital in Bayonne, New Jersey, only after "considerable correspondence and telegrams."[62] Some local authorities remained intransigent. A request by the county hospital to transfer a "Mexican unmarried minor girl" was rejected in a letter stating, "We do not have in the State of New Mexico an institution for the care of tubercular women."[63] We saw that the Globe, Arizona, hospital superintendent initially refused to accept the Garcia children even after the ambulances had departed to take them to the station. When officials of Bates County, Missouri, agreed to receive a forty-eight-year-old man with "far advanced pulmonary tuberculosis," they urged Los Angeles County Hospital to "please bear in mind the following when you make this return. Missouri is covered with alternative layers of mud, ice and slosh. We have no funds with which to assure food and fuel for this family and no hospitalization whatever. Our only possible hope for pneumothorax treatment lies in the possibility of having a case accepted at Mt. Vernon Sanitarium at Mt. Vernon, Missouri, which is overcrowded and refusing all applicants at this time."[64]

And some requests met silence. Los Angeles County Hospital wanted to transfer a "divorced Jewish Polish man, 30 years of age" to Detroit, his legal residence. He had first come to Los Angeles in 1935 to enter the Jewish Consumptive Relief Association in Duarte; the following year he returned to Detroit but was now back in Los Angeles and had recently entered the tuberculosis ward of the county hospital. The case file noted, "We endeavored from August to November, 1936, to get some response from Detroit but received no response to letters or telegrams."[65]

Convincing clients to depart was even more difficult. Tate-Thompson managed to persuade a Long Beach woman with two tubercular children to return to Seattle only after threatening to report her to juvenile authorities and holding two conferences, one involving "all of the agencies in Long Beach."[66] Other cases did not end successfully. As a social worker stated, "We try to send them back home, but they won't go"; many people refused to "return to nothing where they came from."[67] Tate-Thompson concurred, "Caught either in the drought or the flood districts, [migrants] feel they can stand almost anything in California rather than return."[68]

Family issues often intensified resistance. Although Mrs. Gottlieb, a Jewish Social Service Bureau (JSSB) client, had come to Los Angeles from New York to improve her health, her decision followed "an estrangement with her husband." Unwilling to live near him again, she declined to return.[69] A tubercular man who had deserted his wife and children in Chicago similarly rejected the society's offer of transportation home.[70] Conversely, some migrants were loath to rupture ties established since arriving in town. Those who had come with family members were reluctant to leave them. Even the JSSB caseworker doubted it would be "humane" to send an "aged grandmother back to Cleveland, in view of the fact that her two married daughters are living in L.A."[71]

The health concerns that pushed sick people to California also strengthened their determination to remain. Tate-Thompson's December 1938 report described a "very defiant" woman whose husband had tuberculosis. The wife "said that even as sick as the man was, he had improved," and "nobody could make them go back to Missouri if they did not want to go."[72] The following year Tate-Thompson spent "a great deal of time" in "correspondence regarding cases of migrants with tuberculosis. Most of them are new arrivals who have been treated in Eastern and Midwest sanatoria. They claim the doctors told them to come to California. Nearly all of them refuse to return to their legal residence."[73] According to a County Department of Health case file, a woman urged to return to New Brunswick, New Jersey, for care responded that "she had 'froze' in the East long enough and intended to make California her home."[74] Several tubercular clients of the JSSB similarly worried that severe winters would again aggravate their condition.[75] Perhaps one reason Rafael Garcia repeatedly made objections to his family's return is that he shared his wife's doubts about the quality of tuberculosis care in Globe, Arizona.

Trips from California must have been extremely grueling, especially for travelers as sick as Ernesto Garcia. He was hardly unusual. Because authorities were particularly anxious to transport tubercular migrants with no hope of recovery, people with "far advanced" disease represented a sizeable share of the returnees.[76] And many had to go much farther than to Arizona. The Department of Charities, for example, transported one extremely ill tubercular patient to Natchez, Mississippi, another to Pittsburgh, and a third to Helen, West Virginia.[77] Although separate compartments may have eased the travails of some sick passengers, the Garcia case reminds us that plans could proceed even when railroads failed to provide the special accommodations health authorities requested.[78]

Suffering must have continued after returnees reached their destinations. "Unfortunately," Tate-Thompson acknowledged in 1938, the Bureau of Tuberculosis "has gone through the humiliation of having people return, even though the state sanatorium has said they would take them, only to receive word that they did not have a bed, and in the winter the personal misery of these people in the eastern states is very great if they are ill and poor."[79] A social worker in a Los Angeles SRA office recalled that staff members enjoyed considerable discretion about individual cases. Some workers simply wrote to officials in clients' home communities, waited a certain length of time, and then arranged for transportation regardless of whether or not a response had been received.[80] The letters to the Board of Supervisors by Rex Thomson and A. C. Price suggest that very sick patients could be sent in the absence of assurances they would receive adequate care at home. Thomson noted that a sixteen-year-old girl who had been a "full bed patient" in the county hospital would stay in an aunt's house "until arrangements can be made for hospitalization."[81] Price sought a companion not only to "look after" a man during the trip but "also to attend to anything which might arise in connection with taking a sick person into another locality where they may not have everything ready to care for him."[82]

The many people who rejected transportation offers also fared very poorly. Drawing on a California survey conducted in 1936, W. H. Lewis summarized "the lot" of the unemployed non-resident: "There is no room for him even in the poor-house, in the county hospital, or on the so-called dole. He is reduced to the status of a beggar. He must panhandle on the city streets, ask for food from door to door—or starve. . . . There is no method by which he can procure new clothing or needed medical care."[83] The plight of migrants afflicted with tuberculosis must have been particularly grim.

In one way Rafael Garcia was fortunate. As a household head, he escaped the opprobrium directed toward "unattached" men. Despite the phenomenal growth of the number of families on the road, the majority of depression-era migrants were single.[84] Although less likely to be called "tramps" than a generation earlier, they incurred the same wrath. Most congregated in the downtown skid row area, joining the larger, older, homeless male population that had lived there for years; indeed, officials tended to use the terms "transient men" and "homeless men" interchangeably. [85] (Although the number of single, homeless women increased during the 1930s, they still were relatively rare and received little attention from L.A. authorities.)[86]

New Deal programs had little to offer. As one historian writes, most viewed "family breadwinning" as central to "masculine citizenship" and thus disqualified unattached men from benefits.[87] Only the Federal Transient Service accommodated that population; after its termination, most single men had to fend for themselves. When Rafael Garcia indicated that he might remain in Los Angeles, the local State Relief Administration office warned that if he refused to follow his family to Arizona, "his status would be that of an unattached, employable transient man, and he would not be eligible for relief."[88]

The sole city agency serving single men was the Municipal Service Bureau, established in 1928 as a clearinghouse for those seeking assistance from private charities. A 1933 report found that the bureau addressed "the problem of transients in such a way as to protect the interests of the community." Improving the men's well-being apparently was not a priority. The specific objectives were "(1) Prevention of the spread of communicable diseases by promptly isolating the infected men in proper hospitals or clinics; (2) Relieving the community of sick or idle transients by referring those with serious physical or age handicaps to the County Welfare Department, with a view to their being returned to their legal residence; (3) Prevention of crime by giving the men such employment as comes to the attention of the Bureau, and by sending them to work camps."[89] Low funding further restricted the bureau's purview. Although the number of applicants had increased 500 percent during the past four years, its budget had remained constant. As a result, medical examinations were "hasty and primarily organized to detect venereal disease." "Other ailments, such as tuberculosis and organic difficulties," were likely to "slip by unnoticed."[90]

"Unemployable," single men (including the many with tuberculosis) could receive public financial assistance only from the County Department of Charities. Because most had been away from home too long to retain residence, they could not be returned. Instead, they were placed in cheap lodging houses and given meal tickets for use in local restaurants.[91] That practice provoked numerous criticisms, especially from Tate-Thompson. In March 1934 she reported that "many old men, sick and old, who are on the County Welfare" came into her office "protesting over the 14c a day allowance they have for food. The clinic physician had ordered 20c a day. These old men are chronic far-advanced cases, nearly all without teeth and so feeble they can scarcely walk."[92] Her concern, however, was less the health of the men than their lack of supervision. In April she complained that "the lodging house keepers" assumed little responsibility for the "old men who sleep on the roof and brush off dry expectoration into the air."[93] The following month she warned that "these people" could not "be permitted to stay in lodging houses and furnished rooms and roam the streets without it meaning a vast circle which as the years go on cannot be broken."[94] Like many other observers, she accused the men of abusing alcohol and begging.[95] The "great many single men" who were "being lodged in the lodging house districts in L.A.," she wrote in July, did "a great deal of drinking" and therefore "should be taken from the streets." The majority "used tuberculosis as an opportunity to do a great deal of pan-handling."[96]

The following year the county changed its policy. Now single men with long-term health problems were placed in the American House. Affiliated with the Midnight Mission, that facility was located in an industrial area near the railroads. The concrete and steel building, previously used by the Llewellyn Iron Works, housed staff offices, three dining rooms (including a separate one for men with tuberculosis), and large dormitories furnished with steel cots, blankets, sheets, pillows, and bedspreads.[97] Of the 284 men living there in March 1936, 64 had been diagnosed with tuberculosis.[98]

Tubercular clients at American House also protested, though to no avail. After receiving copies of their complaints from county supervisor John Anson Ford, Rex Thomson defended his policy. "You can readily understand," Thomson wrote, that the practice of housing "indigent tubercular men" in "cheap down-town accommodations" was "not conducive to proper segregation, public protection and preventative measures against infection of others." The men's complaint about the adequacy of their diet was "quite untrue." The food was "prescribed by the dietetic staff of the General Hospital"; each man was permitted a "full quart per day" of milk of "Grade 'A' quality." The second complaint, that "a monetary reason was the paramount one involved in the transfer of these men" was "wholly untrue," although Thomson acknowledged "a savings to the County in the present program." The "real reason for the transfer," however, "was the interest of this Department in the men's own welfare as well as that of the public." But Thomson said nothing further about client "welfare." It was "entirely unfair" to the "general public," he continued, "to permit these men to be on the streets, in hotels, restaurants, parks, etc." By "segregating these men in the American House," they were "completely removed from the heavily populated downtown area." Thomson concluded, "This small group of men, when considered in relation to the great host of residents of Los Angeles County and the controllable possibility of the spread of tuberculosis are, in our opinion, quite properly subject to as close segregation, supervision, and control as it is possible for the County of Los Angeles and this Department to provide."[99]

Tate-Thompson soon would find a way to provide that "close segregation, supervision, and control." She too received "a great deal of trouble" from the American House residents. "For the first time in the twenty-five years I have been doing tuberculosis work," she wrote in January 1936, "I have had a deluge of insults hurled at me by these men." She acknowledged that "there probably is some merit to the complaints of the patients." Nevertheless, the men lacked the standing to make demands: "It would seem to me that it has about reached the point where people who have been on relief for the last ten years and who will be on relief for the rest of their lives will have to learn they can not dictate to everybody just exactly what they wish to do." The major complaints of the men who came to her office "have been very largely to the effect that they did not like to get up for breakfast. When they had the food allowance given them in cash, they could sleep until noon. I told them this was not a legitimate complaint and we would not pay any attention to it." Tate-Thompson attributed much of the problem to social reformers who tried to "stir up as much trouble as they can." Hoping "that taxpayers may see what they are called upon to support in the way of human scrap," she urged "everybody" to visit the facility.[100]

Other documents give some credence to the men's complaints. On May 28, 1939, Supervisor Ford received a long letter from a man who had accompanied a Sunday School class to the residence. He saw "the place at its best just after a Saturday morning cleaning. The food appeared to be fine, and well prepared." But the "fireproofed business building" housing the "incapacitated unfortunate men" was unbearable in the summer heat. "By nature of circumstances," the visitor pointed out, "many men must remain 'indoors' these hot days . . . to escape the sun. Of course . . . some of the men cannot very easily move up and down the stairs, or go out into the shade if shade was provided." However, if even a few men "could be induced to go outside the building," those who remained "would be more comfortable because the dormitories would not be so stuffy, 'smelly,' and crowded." The writer acknowledged that he was "interested in economy" but "not at the expense of needless human suffering." Urging the county supervisors to erect a structure to provide shade on the grounds, he pointed out that the county furnished "double shades" for rabbits "on an adjoining lot."[101] Homeless men apparently deserved at least as much.

What disturbed officials more than the suffering of the men was the renewed threat they seemed to pose to the community. As the population of single men soared, the facility became increasingly inadequate, and the county reverted to the practice of placing sick and disabled patients in downtown hotels. "Why do we, a government agency, throw back upon a supposedly unsuspecting public, cases that we know to be potential sources of danger to the public health?" asked E. J. Sneed, the director of county relief in the skid row area. "One branch of government attempts to maintain restaurants and lunch rooms in sanitary condition, while we send them men who are diseased and potential menaces to the public health. . . . Is it not true that many such cases should be quarantined?"[102] Sneed's suggestion was that the county erect barracks on the American House grounds and convert the first floor into additional dormitories.[103]

Tate-Thompson had a far more ambitious solution. We have seen that she had long advocated low-cost sanatoriums to isolate "undeserving" populations as a way to resolve the conflict between the demands of promoting public safety and reducing health care expenditure. Now she seemed to have an opportunity to put that plan into operation. During the late 1930s she obtained the promise of federal funds for a facility for single, tubercular men and began searching for a suitable site. As usual, she justified her actions by stressing the personal characteristics of the group she sought to quarantine: "A great many of the men who have tuberculosis in Los Angeles County and who are now being cared for at public expense are cases that need to be taken out of circulation, not so much because of tuberculosis but because a good many of them are psychopathic cases. Quite a number of them are drug addicts, and the county would be saving money if these men could be segregated."[104] She also noted that many men were "chronic alcoholics" and had contracted venereal disease as well as tuberculosis.[105] In 1938 she announced she had found "an ideal place" for an "800-bed colony for men." The plan would "cost less than caring for them on the outside."[106]

But two problems soon arose. The first stemmed from the primacy of real estate speculation in Southern California. A group of investors planned to build close to the site she had chosen and convinced county officials that "convalescing men recovering from tuberculosis" would drastically lower the value of the land.[107] A state proposal for a $35 pension for handicapped people represented a second problem. As Tate-Thompson acknowledged, there was "no doubt" that most men would "prefer $35 a month to a convalescent colony."[108] Although she hated "to be against anything that might help the tuberculous," the passage of the bill "might make discipline and recovery impossible."[109]

Tate-Thompson next discussed her colony scheme in her last extant monthly report, for March 1941, when she wrote that she had received a promise from the county that she could turn a facility at Acton into a "convalescent colony" with 360 beds. Although the colony would be much smaller than the one she originally had envisioned, it would further her campaign of exclusion: "This will remove the numbers of men who have caused so much trouble from circulating around."[110] Soon afterwards, the county opened a detention facility for tuberculosis patients assumed to need more control than could be provided in hospitals and sanatoriums.

Chapter 8

Fighting TB in Black Los Angeles

Unlike Mexicans, Filipinos, and "inter-state migrants," African Americans could neither be barred from California nor sent home. But they resembled the groups targeted by the early twentieth-century campaign of exclusion in two critical ways. Like Mexicans, African Americans were assumed to have an innate predisposition to tuberculosis. And if they could not be expelled, they could be subjected to various forms of "social exclusion"— the denial of access to a community's major institutions.[1] As an unwanted ethnic minority, black Los Angelenos suffered severely after the 1929 stock market crash. Despite extremely high unemployment rates, very few African Americans gained assistance from local, state, and federal relief programs. Although tuberculosis struck large numbers of blacks, public health programs gave priority to whites.

More than any other L.A. community activism in the 1930s, the African American crusade to expand access to TB care subverted the values underlying public health policy. As in other areas, blacks employed a two-pronged approach—demanding equal treatment and establishing separate institutions.[2] Under the leadership of Dr. Leonard Stovall, community members convinced the local antituberculosis association to direct at least some attention to their needs and launched a successful drive to build their own sanatorium.

The city's black population had grown steadily since the late-nineteenth century, reaching nearly 40,000 by 1930.[3] We have seen that the late-nineteenth century booster campaign spearheaded by the Los Angeles Chamber of Commerce had focused exclusively on Anglo-Saxons, enticing them with the promise of living in an all-white society. Simultaneously, however, African American publicists wooed members of their race. Some gave a special twist to the booster rhetoric. An article entitled "California for Colored Folks" proclaimed Southern California "more adapted for the colored man than any other part of the United States" because the climate was "distinctively African."[4] One local black newspaper declared, "California for ours, Los Angeles and Southern California always, and our people here, the best forevermore."[5] Another wrote that blacks would "find no race problem in Los Angeles, only prosperity."[6] Such messages had great appeal to African Americans in the post-Reconstruction South, and they flocked to the new land.

They were not entirely disappointed. In Los Angeles, everyone could vote, and social interactions with whites were relatively easy. By 1910, more than 35 percent of black families had purchased homes.[7] Ten years later, the black community boasted two-hundred professionals, including sizeable numbers not just of clergymen but also of physicians, dentists, lawyers, social workers, and teachers. Other African Americans owned businesses, many patronized by whites as well as blacks.[8]

But the metropolis was far from the heaven black publicists had promised. In addition to its manifold attractions, the city had a flourishing Ku Klux Klan, restrictive real estate covenants, and segregated swimming pools and schools. Discriminatory hiring practices confined most blacks to service and menial positions. Fully 87 percent of female black workers and 40 percent of male workers were domestic servants in 1930.[9] As we will see, those jobs left African Americans especially vulnerable to the charge that they spread TB germs to whites.

Racism also pervaded the health care system. The *California Eagle*, the city's major black newspaper, explained why Dr. D. N. Arthurton left for Northern California in 1919: "Cramped in his efforts to do surgery in accordance with his ability, not being allowed to use the operating rooms in the various hospitals in Los Angeles, as was his custom in Chicago . . . the doctor transferred his activities to Oakland."[10] Two years later, the paper praised the newly opened Japanese Hospital as the only institution "in this great city" where it was "possible for a Negro Surgeon to have full charge in a major operation."[11] In 1927, the *Eagle* announced that L.A. County Hospital had accepted an African American intern for the first time;[12] an investigation conducted by the paper four years later revealed that the hospital superintendent had assumed that the applicant was white, and that, once his race was revealed, he had been forced to consent to the "most humiliating and disgraceful terms." He could not examine, treat, or attend the delivery of any white women, could not treat any patient "either white or colored" who objected to him because of his race, and had to be "particularly careful to avoid any form or suggestion of dispute or conflict of authority in giving orders to nurses or other employees" concerning patients he had seen.[13]

Patients as well as providers encountered discrimination. When a group of African American physicians established Dunbar Hospital in 1923 (the "height of the black hospital movement"[14]), the *Eagle* encouraged readers to support the twenty-five-bed facility by noting that it filled "a dire need in the Black American colony of Los Angeles, both from the viewpoint of Negro Physicians and Surgeons who are denied the privilege of operating in white institutions; and from the viewpoint of Colored American patients who often do not find an easy entrance into hospitals."[15] An editorial added, "Institutions conducted by the white people might take you, but we must whisper to you that they don't want you."[16] Access to tuberculosis care was extremely limited. Although a 1923 directory listed fourteen tuberculosis hospitals and sanatoriums in and around Los Angeles, only the two county facilities (Olive View and the county hospital) specified that "Negroes" were "admitted."[17]

The long fight to admit blacks to the county nursing school was not only a major early community struggle but also one with enormous implications for African American tuberculosis patients. As a result, it deserves special attention. Nursing schools in the United States first accepted students in 1873; fifty years later, one quarter of all hospitals had established affiliated training schools.[18] Although hospitals advertised the advanced medical training the schools dispensed, their primary function was to provide cheap labor. Students were required to work long hours six days a week. Despite the degradation and drudgery involved, however, the education provided women with one of their few routes to a professional career, and they clamored for admission. The degree was especially prized in the black community where, as one historian writes, nurses traditionally "have enjoyed a level of respect and responsibility unusual in the larger society."[19]

But black women seeking nursing careers encountered overwhelming obstacles. Schools throughout the South admitted only whites. Those in the North typically imposed strict racial quotas; the school at the New England Hospital for Women and Children in Boston, for example, accepted one black and one Jewish student each year.[20] It is thus likely that when the Training School for Nurses at the Los Angeles County Hospital opened in 1895, few observers were surprised that its eight-woman student body was exclusively white.[21]

After the turn of the century, black Americans increasingly demanded nursing education. A few black physicians established separate institutions where women could receive nursing training; simultaneously, other community leaders sought to end discriminatory admissions policies.[22] The L.A. campaign began in 1911. That October, C. H. Whitman, the hospital superintendent, informed the Board of Supervisors that "a colored attorney of this city" had protested that "a young colored woman" had applied to the hospital nursing school but was told that "colored women were not admitted." The lawyer was "considerably exercised over the matter," though he had been "very gentlemanly about it."[23]

The following month the Board of Supervisors received two petitions. The first was signed by eighty-five "officers and nurses of the Training School" who had "heard with alarm of the effort which is being made to open the School to colored girls" and wished to register "their strongest protest against it." "Disclaiming any personal prejudice," they believed the time had "not yet come for the two races to mix on terms of equality." Should the board attempt "to establish this element in the School," the result would be "disastrous to the interests and good standing of the institution," "cause bitterness, hard feeling and strife," "prevent an adequate number of applicants," and "very materially" lower the "*class* of girls seeking admission." The board should refuse to cater "to the wishes of a very small minority."[24] The second petition came from thirty-five "citizens of the County of Los Angeles" protesting Whitman's refusal to admit black applicants.[25]

On April 1, 1912, the board finally issued its decision: African American women would be admitted to the school but housed in a separate building. Although we learn that a mass meeting at New Hope Baptist Church protested the imposition of any form of segregation,[26] the records are silent about the response of whites. We can assume, however, that when the board rescinded its decision to admit African Americans, it did so in response to white objections.

Two events probably encouraged blacks to renew the fight six years later. One was the establishment of a local branch of the National Association for the Advancement of Colored People (NAACP) in 1914.[27] The other was the U.S. entry into World War I. As *Eagle* editor Charlotta A. Bass later wrote, "Negroes who were being called upon to defend their country in conflict with Germany were aroused over the second-class citizenship role forced upon them." Discrimination "was particularly galling at a time when many young men were leaving their homes for battlefields in Europe."[28] The 1917 annual report of the NAACP commented, "If thousands of American black men do fight in this war, joining hands with the hundred thousand or more colored troops [from French Africa] that are fighting for the Allies in Europe, then who can hold from them the freedom that should be theirs in the end?"[29] In June 1918 the NAACP petitioned the board to admit "members of the Negro race to the Training School for Nurses." Other signatories included several African American professional associations, a day nursery, and a federation of women's clubs.[30] A nursing shortage may have encouraged the board to respond favorably. Unable to find an adequate number of nursing graduates, the hospital had begun hiring untrained assistants in January 1917.[31] Understaffing probably became especially severe as nurses increasingly departed for the war front. Although the admission of blacks to the training school would not increase the total number of student workers, the board may have concluded that this was the wrong time to discourage any group of women from joining the profession. In any case, on July 17, 1918, the board ordered the school "to receive colored women for training."[32]

But the struggle was far from over. Twelve days later, Superintendent of Charities Norman R. Martin told the board that he had received a letter from 143 students and graduate nurses at the hospital along with eighteen physicians and interns. They began by reminding him of the nurses' 1911 letter stating "in positive terms that they would neither work with nor live in the environment with colored nurses." The "principal difficulty" had been the lack of "separate quarters which might be used." That problem had not been remedied. And there was an additional issue: "The necessary system of instruction is such that in the senior year colored nurses would be put in direct control of junior and middler [sic] nurses, and such white student nurses would be obliged to take instructions from colored seniors." Martin added, "Personally, I have no prejudice whatever against the colored race." Nevertheless, he pointed out that he had "a long waiting list of white women applicants who desire student training and whom we are unable to accept on account of lack of housing facilities."[33] The *Eagle* condemned the "supreme gall and brazen impudence" of the white nurses, who were "tearing down democracy at home faster than the boys who are fighting for it in the trenches can build it up."[34]

This time the white nurses won only a temporary victory. Shortly after the flu epidemic struck Los Angeles in the fall of 1918, the board suspended its order, noting that the hospital staff had been "employed for long hours" and thus been "under extraordinary strain." The board wished to "prevent further disorganization of the nursing force at the Hospital."[35] Once the crisis passed, however, the order was reinstated, and in March 1919, NAACP attorney E. Burton Ceruti announced that the entering class of the school would include four African American women, Adele E. Kemp, Ethel M. Strotters, Victoria P. Anderson, and Helen P. Gladden.[36]

They would require great courage and strength. In 1931, the *Eagle* reported that black students were housed in separate quarters, "barred from the Alumni Association," and "until recently . . . obliged to receive their diplomas off stage after graduation exercises."[37] Few jobs awaited the graduates. A 1928 article in the *Eagle* complained about "our girls finishing nurse training at the County Hospital with nothing to aspire to in the way of positions in an institution after the positions are filled in Dunbar Hospital."[38] Studies conducted during the late

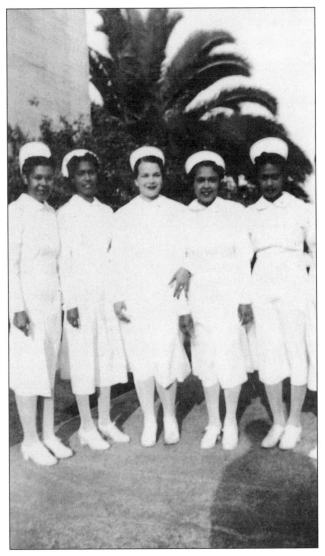

Figure 9. African American nurses at Los Angeles County Hospital in 1940

Courtesy of Photograph Collection, Los Angeles Public Library.

1930s pointed to the discriminatory aspects of the Civil Service examination, required for all jobs at both the county hospital and Olive View Sanatorium.[39]

And discrimination continued after hiring. According to a 1931 *Eagle* article, African American nurses at the hospital were required to eat in "a segregated corner, partitioned off from the main dining room," could use the nurses' tennis courts "only one afternoon a week," and were not permitted to attend the nurses' annual picnic. Two years later the paper noted that when the hospital posted the board's executive order abolishing separate dining rooms, "it was read with disfavor by the white nurses" and "the colored nurses were warned not to eat in the general dining room."[40] A "report was also broadcast that on one occasion stones or bricks were hurled at the nurses as they left the building."[41] An Occidental College student wrote in 1933 that "black and white nurses employed in the county hospital did the same types of work, except that the colored nurses are not left in charge or given executive positions where they would have authority over white women."[42]

We can only speculate about how the hostility directed toward African American nurses translated into the quality of care white social workers, nurses, and doctors delivered to patients. Were African Americans with tuberculosis less likely than whites to be transferred from the hospital to Olive View? Where they more likely to be relegated to inferior rest homes? Did African Americans encounter the same kind of abuse Carlos Bulosan reported at the county hospital? Although we cannot answer those questions, the *Eagle* prominently reported any charges of mistreatment from hospital staff. In 1934, for example, a white nurse was "said to have slapped a colored patient . . . because he addressed her as 'lady' instead of nurse."[43] A 1939 banner headline announced that an African American father removed his nineteen-year-old son from the hospital because a doctor had beaten him.[44]

Tuberculosis was the focus of the second major black health movement in Los Angeles. The leader, Dr. Leonard Stovall, had arrived from Atlanta, Georgia, at the age of eight in 1896.[45] Despite that city's thriving black middle class and prominent black colleges, his family would have had ample reasons to leave. Discrimination relegated most blacks to the most arduous and lowest-paying jobs. The public schools available to African American children were grossly deficient. And the state poll tax deprived most African Americans of the right to vote. Three years after Stovall's departure, a white mob lynched a black man. A 1906 race riot left black neighborhoods devastated and several African Americans dead.[46]

If Stovall kept track of events in his native city, he also would have learned about the panic that engulfed the white community during the early twentieth century about the presumed propensity of black servants and washerwomen to spread tuberculosis. "We are ever subject to the death-dealing micro-organism at their hands," one white physician wrote. "They daily traverse our every pathway, enter every department of our homes as servants, directly, if you please, from the contaminated and polluted huts, cabins, hovels, slums, and dives, handling every vestige of linen, clothing, furniture, bric-a-brac, books, etc., in our living apartments, dining rooms, pantries, kitchens, and dairies."[47] But Atlanta also was the

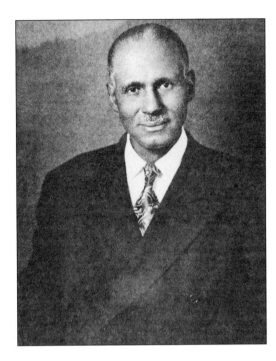

Figure 10. Dr. Leonard
Stovall in his later years
Courtesy of Photograph Collection,
Los Angeles Public Library.

site of a major black antituberculosis association, which successfully collaborated
with white leaders to address the ravages of the disease in the black community.[48]
As a young doctor in another city with a large number of African American domestic servants, Stovall may have looked to that society for inspiration.

A few days after his death in 1956, the *Eagle* wrote:

> Stovall's life was full of "firsts." He was the first of his race to graduate
> from the Los Feliz Grammar School, Hollywood High School and to
> receive a medical degree from the University of California. He was also
> the first member of his race to become a staff member of the Los Angeles
> County General Hospital and a member of the House of Delegates of the
> California Medical Society. He was the first person to conduct a tuber-
> culosis survey on the eastside of Los Angeles and . . . was the founder
> and president of the Outdoor Life and Health Association.[49]

Surviving records shed light on the determination and energy the last two
accomplishments involved. In July 1934 Edythe Tate-Thompson, the director
of the State Bureau of Tuberculosis, discussed a meeting with Stovall and a
physician from a "colored Health Center on East 28th Street" which had been
"started in the midst of the negro district in Los Angeles for the purpose of raising
the standard of health of the colored people in this district, also endeavoring to

do some educational work among them." Tate-Thompson had told Stovall that she "was very anxious to help any colored group who wished to operate their own clinic as against mixing them in with poor whites" and she described "the very fine piece of work that has been done in the Central Harlem District in New York where Federal aid under the Emergency Relief Act was secured and a survey conducted among all families that were on relief." Seeking to obtain the support of the director of the State Department of Public Health for the survey, Tate-Thompson invoked the most common white rationale for addressing the high tuberculosis rates among African Americans: "I feel that it is particularly necessary that such a piece of work be done at this time because these colored people come in contact with white people more than almost any other group in Los Angeles because they are in house service, porters, waiters and chefs and because of their ambition, they are rapidly getting into a great many other occupations, such as barbers and cosmetitians."[50]

Although Tate-Thompson continued to endorse the survey in November, she noted that local officials were far less enthusiastic. The project had angered both Dr. George Parish, the director of the City Department of Health, and Dr. Harry Cohn, the director of the Tuberculosis Division. Tate-Thompson's own rationale now shifted, from fear of the spread of germs to fear of the power of the black community. If "large groups of colored people in Los Angeles, through the colored churches and organizations," learned that the project had been stalled, "there might be trouble."[51]

But that argument was not enough to sustain Tate-Thompson's support, and it soon faltered. After visiting Los Angeles in August 1935, she wrote, "The project requested by the colored people has been held in abeyance because of the fact that it will have to be done in conjunction with the city health department." She saw "no reason why the city health department and the Bureau of Tuberculosis should cooperate on a project for colored people. The city health department is understaffed and can not even take care of the patients who come to the clinic."[52] The implication was that the department's patients were overwhelmingly white and that its purview did not extend to the black community. Tate-Thompson did not mention the survey again until March 1939, when she remarked, "There is still a great need for a program among Negroes in Los Angeles City and County, and the colored people themselves have asked repeatedly for assistance, which I have been unable to give."[53]

The city anti-TB society was slightly more responsive to Stovall. Like similar groups throughout the United States,[54] the Los Angeles Tuberculosis and Health Association defined itself as a white organization. In the spring of 1933, the group's executive secretary noted he was working with the "colored physicians who were getting together thru Dr. Leonard Stovall."[55] It was important to encourage the formation of a "colored auxiliary" because the "colored group" was "more susceptible to tuberculosis" than others.[56] By the early 1930s, that belief was well entrenched among whites. One of the most prominent early proponents had been Frederick Ludwig Hoffman, whose 1896 *Race Traits and Tendencies of the American Negro* offered statistical "proof" that the high tuberculosis morbidity and mortality rates of African Americans stemmed from innate physical weakness. "Given the same conditions of life for two races," he concluded, "the one of Aryan descent will prove the superior, solely on account of its ancient inheritance of virtue and transmitted qualities which are determining factors in the struggle for race supremacy."[57] A founder of the National Association for the Study and Prevention of Tuberculosis and later vice president of the Prudential Insurance Company of Newark, New Jersey, Hoffman spread those ideas throughout the country. His views also encountered vehement opposition, most famously from W.E.B. Du Bois.[58] A 1931 *Eagle* editorial wrote, "So long as America insists on discriminating against the Negro in industry, paying him lower wages and otherwise forcing his living standard down that long must the Negro live in disease infested neighborhoods, subsist on inferior necessities and thus invite the ravages of disease and death."[59]

In February 1935, the executive secretary of the local anti-TB organization noted that the National Negro Health Week would begin the following month and that he was "cooperating with the local committee to make this campaign educational and of value to the community's negro population."[60] Established by Booker T. Washington at the Tuskegee Institute (now Tuskegee University) in 1915, the National Negro Health Week was an annual event offering a broad array of health education programs throughout the county. The 1932 opening of the Office of Negro Health Week under the United States Public Health Service represented, according to one historian, "a milestone in the history of American public health." For the "first time since the Freedmen's Bureau," the "federal government institutionalized black health work within the federal bureaucracy."[61] L.A. plans for the 1933 observation included exhibits, lectures, mass meetings, and even a prize for the best student essay on black health.[62]

Lobbying by black activists and doctors appears to have been necessary to convince the Los Angeles Tuberculosis and Health Association to participate in further biracial activities. In January 1938, the executive secretary reported that both the Los Angeles Urban League and the Negro Medical Association had written "urging the adoption of a program of tuberculosis control among Negroes."[63] Founded in 1921, the L.A. branch of the Urban League quickly took its place alongside the NAACP as a leading activist group.[64] The organization of black physicians, the National Medical Association protested segregation in health care throughout the United States.[65] The letters sent by both groups must have had some effect because in August the board of directors of the anti-TB society previewed "an all-Negro motion picture, 'Let My People Live,'" to be made "available throughout the "Negro community."[66] The report for 1938 noted that the film was "so enthusiastically received" that "the Association was asked to show it again and again."[67] In addition, the board agreed to donate $350 toward two activities initiated by Dr. Stovall, a seminar for "Negro Physicians in this community" and a "special case finding program" to be "conducted in a selected Negro area."[68] Like Tate-Thompson, the board defended the assistance to African Americans by highlighting the advantages to whites. The executive committee stated, "Because of the high incidence of tuberculosis among Negroes and the high proportion of these people engaged in domestic and personal service," the seminar and survey "would prove of benefit to the entire community."[69]

Because Stovall envisioned his sanatorium as a self-help project, he could devote his energy to galvanizing the black community rather than soliciting white assistance. "As with all great undertakings," the *Eagle* later wrote, the rest home (as it soon was called) "began with the dream of one man." Stovall's "first moves came at a time when great insurance houses and medical authorities were just concocting the poisonous notion that Negroes are particularly susceptible to tuberculosis."[70] The earliest mention of those "moves" was a 1916 article reporting, "Dr. Leonard Stovall and several visiting physicians addressed the Forum on the need of a Sanitarium."[71] (Established by the First African Methodist Episcopal Church in 1903, the Los Angeles Sunday Forum quickly became a major community institution, offering a place where opinions could be voiced on various topics.)[72] One of those "visiting" physicians was Dr. Shuman, a founder of the Jewish Consumptive Relief Association Sanatorium. The article concluded, "The Jewish people have a fine institution at Duarte and they built it by small contributions from their own people of from 25c to $1 and more, the rich people did not help much, it was done by the wage earners. We can do as much."[73] In 1922 the *Eagle* noted that Stovall was investigating a possible site in Mexico;[74] a 1923 benefit raised money.[75] Then the reports stop, however, suggesting Stovall abandoned the project for several years.

Various factors may help explain why he was far more successful in the 1930s. During the past decade he had risen to a position of eminence in the medical community, the city's African American population had dramatically increased, and various all-black enterprises had been established. In addition, the misery inflicted by the depression had helped to revive community activism, which had waned during the late 1920s.[76] And the policy of substituting rest-home care for stays in Olive View (harmful though it may have been to patients) offered one major advantage. If Stovall's facility passed inspection, he could obtain the $3 subsidy from the state for each patient.

But he faced enormous obstacles. By 1934, when he organized the Outdoor Life and Health Association to launch the new enterprise, half of all black Los Angelenos were unemployed.[77] Nevertheless, during the next six years, the *Eagle* reported growing community support as well as a vast array of fund-raising activities, including raffles, balls, beauty contests, floral shows, carnivals, track meets, concerts, and subscription drives.[78] The paper's endorsement also was critical. As Charlotta Bass remarked, "the press and the pulpit" were "the two main centers of community consciousness."[79] A staunch advocate of black businesses, Bass continually exhorted her readers to rally around Stovall's project. "Because the Tubercular Rest Home" was "purely a race enterprise," she "hoped that every Negro in Los Angeles" would "make some contribution."[80] Bass's early history may have bolstered her enthusiasm. Like so many other Los Angelenos, she had arrived as a health seeker. She later recalled that she came to Los Angeles in 1910 "for a two-year health-recuperation stay." A physician had "advised" her to "spend as much time as possible in the sunshine."[81] Perhaps memories of her own illness made her especially supportive of the rest home. She noted that it promised to address "the particular needs of tuberculosis patrons among Negroes as well as the lack of accommodation for them in most local private and public hospitals."[82] A nurse quoted in the *Eagle* pointed to the advantages the facility could offer members of her profession: "I don't see very much opportunity for advancement of colored nurses at the Los Angeles [County] Hospital". Institutions like the rest home would serve "as the way out and upward for the colored nurse who wants to do more than tend patients at the bedside."[83]

When the sixteen-bed facility opened in June 1940, Tate-Thompson dispensed her customary disdain. The rest home was "little," and she regretted "that the colored people could not find a better site." The building was "located in a wash between a hog ranch and a dairy."[84]

But the new facility had a very different meaning to the black community. The *Eagle* pronounced the rest home an "outstanding achievement and a progressive step toward the alleviation of human suffering."[85] Here black doctors could practice without submitting to the "most humiliating and disgraceful terms" the county hospital imposed. Black nurses could rise to supervisory positions. And black patients could receive essential care without sacrificing their dignity. Placing the well-being of black Los Angelenos at the center of its mission, the facility directly challenged the attitudes of public health officials and advocates. Unlike Take-Thompson, most visitors who toured the building after the inaugural ceremony were "highly impressed."[86]

Epilogue

Tuberculosis is again on the rise. Worldwide, two billion people are infected with the tubercle bacillus each year; nine million of them develop active disease.[1] Although the 1946 introduction of streptomycin made TB cures possible, some new strains resist all drugs in the medical armamentarium.[2] The disease continues to impoverish households and devastate quality of life. In India, more than 30,000 children annually withdraw from school because their parents suffer from tuberculosis, and approximately 100,000 affected women are abandoned by their families.[3] The great majority of cases occur in the global South, especially where HIV leaves the population vulnerable to other afflictions. "We cannot win the battle against AIDS if we do not also fight TB," warns Nelson Mandela. "TB is too often a death sentence for people with AIDS."[4] Tuberculosis incidence increases especially rapidly in sub-Saharan Africa, but many victims lack access to effective treatment.[5]

In the United States, immigrants bear the brunt of the disease. Despite a decline among the native-born population since 1992, the TB rate among immigrants continues to increase.[6] Recent California studies document the suffering of Mexican farm workers, who provide the country with good food but cannot afford to eat well themselves. Because adequate nutrition is essential to build resistance, many live with tuberculosis and other serious, chronic maladies; very few, however, have access to health care.[7]

As in the 1920s and 1930s, tuberculosis helps to define who should be considered a member of U.S. society and who should be treated as an outsider. Contemporary reports thus have a familiar ring. Once again, experts highlight the high TB prevalence among immigrants from Mexico and Asia and fault them for importing the disease.[8] Anti-immigration groups emphasize that point, especially in diatribes against undocumented immigrants. A widely reprinted 2005 article asserts that "the illegal alien . . . is assumed healthy even though he and his illegal alien wife and children were never examined for contagious diseases." Nevertheless, "many illegal aliens harbor fatal diseases that American medicine fought and vanquished long ago, such as drug-resistant tuberculosis."[9] After the massive demonstrations of spring 2006, the *New York Times* reported that the marches had intensified "worries that illegal immigrants from Mexico brought with them crime, financial burdens, national security risks, cultural disintegration, and even disease like drug-resistant tuberculosis."[10]

A July 2005 *Los Angeles Times* article by Solomon Moore bears a striking resemblance to a 1938 report by the Los Angeles Department of Charities about tuberculosis in an extended Mexican immigrant family. That report, we recall, obfuscated the distinction between latent infection and active disease, while stressing the high number of cases among the descendants of a Mexican immigrant. Moore's article begins with a discussion of nine-month-old Jason Montanes, whose mother is quoted as saying, " 'Jason started coughing real bad five months ago. I took him to Kaiser a couple of times, but they kept telling me he had a cold.' " Finally, he was diagnosed with tuberculosis. "He probably caught it from his uncle," the article continues, "who had the rattling cough of someone with advanced TB. Like many people from immigrant families, the uncle didn't seek help until he was really sick. Now, eight of Jason's close relatives, who live either with him or nearby, are infected, including his mother, his father, and his immigrant grandparents. Only Jason and the uncle, however, have active cases. Jason still has a mild cough and is probably still contagious."[11]

Moore might have emphasized the negligence of the doctors or the diligence of the mother, who insisted on bringing the baby back to Kaiser, despite physician indifference. Instead, he focuses on the uncle who, "like many" immigrants, disregarded his early symptoms. Moore fails to note that fears of being reported to authorities encourage growing numbers of undocumented immigrants to delay care.[12] Nor does he mention that, with adequate care and decent living standards, few cases of infection would progress to active disease. But Moore does stress the danger the family poses to the rest of society, quoting a conservative columnist, "If anyone needs another reason to oppose illegal immigration, how about the spread of a deadly communicable disease."

The cost of immigrant health care also continues to receive lavish attention. Passed in 1994, California's Proposition 187 denied all public services to undocumented immigrants; although it could not withstand legal challenge, similar bills have been proposed in several other states.[13] The title of CNN's Lou Dobbs show in April 2005 warned, "Illegal Aliens Putting Strain on Hospitals." Because immigrants are concentrated in the low-paid, nonunionized, contingent labor force, they are disproportionately represented among the uninsured population; many thus enter the health-care system only for emergency treatment. Dobbs warned that hospital emergency rooms are being "invaded" by immigrants "all over the country." Just as Tate-Thompson argued that the large number of Mexicans and Filipinos in tuberculosis wards deprived whites of institutional beds, so Dobbs charged that the "invasion of illegal aliens into our hospital emergency rooms" leaves "thousands of American citizens without care." Ignoring the many causes of rising health-care costs, his program concluded that the expense of the care delivered to immigrants was "overwhelming the system." The "tax burden" was "so great" that counties throughout the nation were compelled "to cut back and just not offer the services." The problem was especially acute in California, where "84 hospitals have closed, overwhelmed by free health care to illegal aliens." Los Angeles County annually spends $200 million on unpaid ambulance bills alone.[14]

According to the *New York Times*, hospitals are reluctant to give uninsured immigrants long-term care, as well as emergency services. Some find ways to discharge chronically ill immigrants prematurely. In a move eerily reminiscent of the 1930s repatriation program of the Los Angeles County Department of Charities, a few "have taken unusual steps, including putting nurses on planes to fly the patients back to their own countries."[15]

Echoes of the past also can be found in the arguments public health advocates routinely employ. We justify prenatal programs by citing statistics demonstrating that an ounce of prevention is worth a pound of cure. We try to save county health-care programs by pointing out that the waiter who serves the Caesar salad in affluent neighborhoods depends on those programs to cure his infection. And we demand greater U.S. responsiveness to the global tuberculosis epidemic by noting that the disease is never more than a flight away.

In the current political climate, it might seem particularly difficult to imagine persuasive arguments that do not invoke the self-interest of privileged Americans. But even as we employ those arguments, we might acknowledge their negative consequences. The crude cost-benefit analyses presented by early twentieth-century anti-TB societies added to the perception that patients who were too sick to return to the labor force had no social value. Assertions about the need to establish sanatoriums to segregate the most contagious patients intensified fears about those remaining in the community. A preoccupation with expedience today has similar disadvantages—heightening hostility toward the vulnerable populations that public health is most committed to serve and undermining efforts to articulate a broad vision of collective responsibility.

During the Great Depression, hundreds of relatives wrote to Franklin and Eleanor Roosevelt, begging for care for sick and disabled children. Most letters sought to demonstrate special worth: the men were honest and reliable workers, the women adhered to the cultural definition of good mothers, and the offspring displayed unusual abilities. One letter, however, was unique. "Please don't throw this letter in the Wast Basket and let that settle it," the woman wrote. Her grandson was "a Colored boy But he is Human and one God is over all."[16] Especially at a time when religious appeals often rest on a much narrower sense of human worth, it is urgent to remember the injunction to regard every life as equally precious. Only when we acknowledge our membership in a global community will we be able to extirpate tuberculosis. Rather than erecting higher and higher barriers against "outsiders," we must improve living standards and distribute effective public health programs both at home and abroad.

Notes

The following abbreviations are used in the notes:

CDW   Charles Dwight Willard Collection, Huntington Library, San Marino, California.

GLAVCB   Greater Los Angeles Visitors and Convention Bureau Collection, Urban Archives Center, Oviatt Library, California State University, Northridge.

GPC   George Pigeon Clements Papers, Collection 118, Department of Special Collections, Charles E. Young Research Library, UCLA.

JAF   John Anson Ford Collection, Huntington Library, San Marino, California.

JFSS   Jewish Family Service Society of Los Angeles Collection, Urban Archives Center, Oviatt Library, California State University, Northridge.

HSC   History and Special Collections, UCLA Louise M. Darling Biomedical Library, Los Angeles.

LACBS   Files of the Los Angeles County Board of Supervisors, Hall of Administration, Los Angeles.

LAUL   Los Angeles Urban League Records, Collection 203, Department of Special Collections, Charles E. Young Research Library, UCLA.

MLS   Diaries of Margaret Love Smith, in the possession of Cathryn Griffith, 200 Commonwealth Ave., Boston, Mass.

MSF   Diary of Martha Shaw Farnsworth, Martha Farnsworth Collection, no. 28, Kansas State Historical Society, Topeka, Kansas.

NACP   National Archives, College Park, Maryland.

NAW   National Archives, Washington, D.C.

OHP   Oral History Program, California State University, Fullerton.

RCC   Records of the Chamber of Commerce, Special Collections, Doheny Library, University of Southern California, Los Angeles.

TMR   "Tuberculosis—Monthly Reports," California State Archives, Sacramento. [Typewritten reports by Edythe Tate-Thompson, Director of the Bureau of Tuberculosis.]

Introduction

1. Louis Adamic, *Laughing in the Jungle: The Autobiography of an Immigrant in America* (New York: Harper and Brothers, 1932), p. 21.
2. D. R. Pattee, "The Land of Sunshine," *Land of Sunshine*, v. 1, no. 1 (June 1894): 13.
3. W. C. Patterson, "Why Am I Here?" *Land of Sunshine*, v. 2, no. 2 (Jan. 1895): 38.
4. Quoted in John Baur, *Health Seekers of Southern California, 1870–1900* (San Marino, Calif.: Huntington Library, 1959), pp. 34–35.
5. Helen Raitt and Mary Collier Wayne, *We Three Came West* (San Diego: Tofua Press, 1974), p. 131.
6. Adamic, *Laughing in the Jungle*, pp. 293, 259.
7. Henry A. Strauss, "B'nai B'rith Lodge News," *B'nai B'rith Messenger*, Feb. 14, 1913.

8. The major histories of tuberculosis in the United States on which I draw include Barbara Bates, *Bargaining for Life: A Social History of Tuberculosis, 1876–1938* (Philadelphia: University of Pennsylvania Press, 1992); Georgina D. Feldberg, *Disease and Class: Tuberculosis and the Shaping of Modern North American Society* (New Brunswick, N.J.: Rutgers University Press, 1995); Barron H. Lerner, *Contagion and Confinement: Controlling Tuberculosis along the Skid Row* (Baltimore: Johns Hopkins University Press, 1998); Katherine Ott, *Fevered Lives: Tuberculosis in American Culture since 1870* (Cambridge, Mass.: Harvard University Press, 1996); Sheila M. Rothman, *Living in the Shadow of Death: Tuberculosis and the Social Experience of Illness in American History* (New York: Basic Books, 1994).

9. See especially Ott, *Fevered Lives*, and Rothman, *Living in the Shadow of Death*.

Chapter 1   Pestilence in the Promised Land

1. Quoted in Robert J. Lifton, *Super Power Syndrome: America's Apocalyptic Confrontation with the World* (New York: Thunder's Mountain Press/Nation Books, 2003), p. 127.

2. See Barbara Bates, *Bargaining for Life: A Social History of Tuberculosis, 1876–1938* (Philadelphia: University of Pennsylvania Press, 1992), pp. 27–28; Katherine Ott, *Fevered Lives: Tuberculosis in American Culture since 1870* (Cambridge, Mass.: Harvard University Press, 1996), pp. 39–40; Sheila M. Rothman, *Living in the Shadow of Death: Tuberculosis and the Social Experience of Illness in American History* (New York: Basic Books, 1994), pp. 131–75.

3. See Rothman, *Living in the Shadow of Death*, pp. 133–34.

4. Benjamin Cummings Truman, *Homes and Happiness in the Golden State of California: Being a Description of the Empire State of the Pacific Coast: Its Inducements to Native and Foreign-Born Emigrants; Its Productiveness of Soil and Its Productions; Its Vast Agricultural Resources; Its Healthfulness of Climate and Equability of Temperature; and Many Other Facts for the Information of the Homeseeker and Tourist*, 3rd ed. (San Francisco: H. S. Crocker and Co., 1885), p. 51, quoted in David M. Wrobel, *Promised Lands: Promotion, Memory, and the Creation of the American West* (Lawrence, Kans.: University Press of Kansas, 2002), p. 39.

5. "Southern California Resorts," *Land of Sunshine*, v. 1, no. 1 (June 1894): 3.

6. Richard Gird, "Beet Culture in Southern California," *Land of Sunshine*, v. 1, no. 1 (June 1894): 17.

7. I. M. Holt, *The Great Interior Fruit Belt and Sanitarium of Southern California* (Riverside, Calif.: Press and Horticulturist Establishment, 1885).

8. Quoted in John E. Baur, *The Health Seekers of Southern California, 1870–1900* (San Marino, Calif.: Huntington Library, 1959), p. 119.

9. M. Y. Beach, "Southern California from a Health-Seeker's Point of View," *Land of Sunshine*, v. 1, no. 1 (Oct. 1894): 101.

10. "Living on Climate," *Land of Sunshine*, v. 1, no. 5 (Oct. 1894): 98.

11. Horace Edwards, "A Southern California Specialty," *Land of Sunshine*, v. 1, no. 3 (Aug. 1894): 61.

12. Frank Wiggins, "Some Big Things," *Land of Sunshine*, v. 2, no. 2 (Jan. 1895): 36.

13. George F. Weeks, *California Copy* (Washington, D.C.: Washington College Press, 1928), p. 30.

14. Weeks, *California Copy*, p. 90.

15. Weeks, *California Copy*, p. 49.

16. See Emily K. Abel, *Suffering in the Land of Sunshine: A Los Angeles Illness Narrative* (New Brunswick, N.J.: Rutgers University Press, 2006).

17. Erving Goffman, *Stigma: Notes on the Management of Spoiled Identity* (New York: Simon and Schuster, 1963), p. 7.

18. See Abel, *Suffering in the Land of Sunshine*.

19. He later established the Frank Wiggins Trade School, now Los Angeles Trade Technical College.

20. Leonard Pitt and Dale Pitt, *Los Angeles A to Z: An Encyclopedia of the City and County* (Berkeley: University of California Press, 1997), p. 546.

21. Charles Dwight Willard, *A History of the Chamber of Commerce of Los Angeles, California, from Its Foundation, September 1888 to the Year 1900* (Los Angeles: Kingsley-Barnes & Neuner, 1899), p. 126.

22. John Steven McGroarty, *History of Los Angeles County* (Chicago: American Historical Society, 1923), vol. 1, p. 354.

23. See D. Freeman, "A Unique Institution," *Land of Sunshine*, v. 2, no. 2 (Jan. 1895): 33.

24. *The Members' Annual, Containing Information about the Los Angeles Chamber of Commerce, Twelfth Year* (Los Angeles: Board of Directors of the Los Angeles Chamber of Commerce, 1900), 57, Box 82, RCC.

25. C. D. Willard, "The New Editor," *Land of Sunshine*, v. 2, no. 1 (Dec. 1894): 12.

26. Charles F. Lummis, *A Tramp across the Continent* (New York: Charles Scribner's Sons, 1925), pp. 1–2.

27. Lummis, *Tramp*, p. 7.

28. Lummis, *Tramp*, p. 15.

29. See Kevin Starr, *Inventing the Dream: California through the Progressive Era* (New York: Oxford University Press, 1985), pp. 132–47.

30. See Baur, *The Health Seekers of Southern California*; Rothman, *Living in the Shadow of Death*; Tom Zimmerman, "Paradise Promoted: Boosterism and the L. A. Chamber of Commerce," *California History*, v. 65 (Winter 1985): 22–33.

31. See Tim Cresswell, *The Tramp in America* (London: Reaktion Books, 2001). The classic description of a moral panic is Stanley Cohen, *Folk Devils and Moral Panic* (London: MacGibbon and Kee, 1972).

32. Emil Bogen, *Surgeon Errant: The Life and Writings of William Henry Bucher, 1874–1934* (Los Angeles: The Angelus Press, 1935), p. 5.

33. See Virginia Scharff, "Mobility, Women, and the West," in *Over the Edge: Remapping the American West*, ed. Valerie J. Matsumoto and Blake Allmendinger (Berkeley: University of California Press, 1999), p. 167.

34. Ernest A. Sweet, "Interstate Migration of Tuberculous Persons, Its Bearing on the Public Health, with Special Reference to the States of Texas and New Mexico," *Public Health Reports*, v. 30, no. 15 (April 9, 1915): 1066.

35. See Cresswell, *Tramp in America*, pp. 110–20; John C. Schneider, "Tramping Workers, 1890–1920: A Subcultural View," in *Walking to Work: Tramps in America, 1890–1935*, ed. Eric H. Monkkonen (Lincoln: University of Nebraska Press, 1984), p. 219.

36. *Annual Report of Department of Health of the City of Los Angeles, California, for the Year Ended June 30, 1917* (Los Angeles: Department of Health, 1917), p. 34.

37. Minutes of the Los Angeles Chamber of Commerce, Dec. 11, 1895, Minutes of Meetings, 1895–97, RCC.

38. See Todd Depastino, *Citizen Hobo: How a Century of Homelessness Shaped America* (Chicago: University of Chicago Press, 2003), p. 12; Eric H. Monkkonen,

"Regional Dimensions of Tramping, North and South, 1880–1910," in *Walking to Work: Tramps in America, 1890–1935*, ed. Monkkonen (Lincoln: University of Nebraska Press, 1984), p. 193; Paul T. Ringenbach, *Tramps and Reformers, 1873–1916: The Discovery of Unemployment in New York* (Westport, Conn.: Greenwood Press, 1973), pp. 3–79.

39. *The Express*, April 2, 1897.
40. Los Angeles *Herald*, Aug. 19, 1903.
41. Los Angeles *Herald*, Aug. 19, 1903.
42. Eric H. Monkkonen, "Introduction," in *Walking to Work: Tramps in America, 1890–1935*, ed. Monkkonen (Lincoln: University of Nebraska Press, 1984), p. 8.
43. Monkkonen, "Introduction," pp. 13–14; Schneider, "Tramping Workers," pp. 212–34.
44. See Depastino, *Citizen Hobo*, p. 61; Paul Groth, *Living Downtown: The History of Residential Hotels in the United States* (Berkeley: University of California Press, 1994), pp. 131–67; Kenneth L. Kusmer, *Down and Out, On the Road: The Homeless in American History* (New York: Oxford University Press, 2002), pp. 148–51; Schneider, "Tramping Workers," p. 219; Richard Steven Street, *Beasts of the Field: A Narrative History of California Farmworkers, 1769–1913* (Stanford, Calif.: Stanford University Press, 2004), pp. 527–571.
45. Street, *Beasts of the Field*, p. 537.
46. Street, *Beasts of the Field*, p. 547.
47. D. C. Barber, "The Care of Tuberculous Patients at the Los Angeles County Hospital," *Southern California Practitioner*, v. 24, no. 1 (Jan. 1909): 24.
48. *Southern California Practitioner*, v. 24, no. 4 (April 1909): 212.
49. See George H. Kress, "Some Maxims for Tuberculosis Patients," *Southern California Practitioner*, v. 24, no. 2 (Feb. 1909): 70–78.
50. "A Tuberculosis Helping Station or Dispensary for Indigent Consumptives," *Southern California Practitioner*, v. 21, no. 4 (April 1906): 192.
51. *California State Board of Health Monthly Bulletin*, v. 1, no. 6 (Nov. 1905): 44.
52. "A Tuberculosis Helping Station," p. 192.
53. Depastino, *Citizen Hobo*, pp. 69–70.
54. Depastino, *Citizen Hobo*, p. 70.
55. MSF. I discuss Martha's early life as well as her experiences after leaving California in *Hearts of Wisdom: American Women Caring for Kin, 1850–1940* (Cambridge, Mass.: Harvard University Press, 2000).
56. MSF, Dec. 19, 1982.
57. MSF, Jan. 10, 1893; Jan. 15, 1893; Jan. 17, 1893.
58. MSF, Jan. 8, 1893.
59. MSF, Feb. 18, 1893.
60. MSF, Feb. 26, 1893.
61. MSF, Jan. 16, 1893.
62. MSF, Feb. 10, 1893.
63. MSF, Feb. 8, 1893.
64. MSF, March 21, 1893.
65. MSF, April 14, 1893.
66. MSF, March 27, 1893.
67. MSF, April 9, 1893.
68. MSF, April 13, 1893.
69. MSF, May 8, 1893.
70. MSF, June 11, 1893.

71. MSF, June 16, 1893.
72. MSF, June 17, 1893.
73. MSF, June 26, 1893.
74. MSF, July 3, 1893.
75. MSF, July 4, 1893.
76. MSF, July 22, 1893.
77. MSF, July 15, 1893.
78. MSF, July 17, 1893.
79. MSF, July 27, 1893.
80. MSF, Aug. 1, 1893.
81. MSF, Aug. 2, 1893.
82. MSF, Oct. 26, 1893.
83. On the gender composition of health travel during the early nineteenth century, see Conevery Bolton Valenčius, "Gender and the Economy of Health on the Santa Fe Trail," *OSIRIS*, v. 19 (2004): 79–92.
84. Quoted in Rothman, *Living in the Shadow of Death*, p. 168.
85. "Report of Investigation into Tuberculosis Records at Los Angeles County Hospital, 1912," in *Report of the California Tuberculosis Commission of the State Board of Health, Sacramento, California* (Sacramento: State Printing Office, 1914), p. 42.
86. JFSS.
87. Charles Dwight Willard to Harriet Edgar Willard, Nov. 17, 1886, CDW.
88. MSF, May 1893.
89. Francis Marion Pottenger, *The Fight against Tuberculosis: An Autobiography* (New York: Henry Schuman, 1952).
90. Interview with Lynne Roberts, July 13, 2006.
91. See Abel, *Suffering in the Land of Sunshine*.
92. Lucy Sprague Mitchell, *Two Lives: The Story of Wesley Clair Mitchell and Myself* (New York: Simon and Schuster, 1953).
93. Mitchell, *Two Lives*, p. 114.
94. Baur, *The Health Seekers of Southern California*, p. 58; Pitt and Pitt, *Los Angeles, A to Z*, p. 468.
95. Mitchell, *Two Lives*, p. 104.
96. See Joyce Antler, *Lucy Sprague Mitchell: The Making of a Modern Woman* (New Haven: Yale University Press, 1987), pp. 50–88.
97. MSF, March 3, 1893.
98. MSF, June 29, 1893.
99. MSF, July 17, 1893.
100. Quoted in Antler, *Two Lives*, p. 34.
101. MSF, Nov. 28, 1892.
102. Mitchell, *Two Lives*, p. 100.
103. Mitchell, *Two Lives*, p. 108.
104. MSF, Dec. 18, 1892.
105. MSF, Dec. 25, 1892.
106. MSF, Jan. 1, 1893.
107. Quoted in Antler, *Two Lives*, p. 32.
108. Mitchell, *Two Lives*, p. 110.
109. Mitchell, *Two Lives*, p. 105.
110. MSF, Dec. 8, 1889.
111. MSF, Dec. 9, 1889.

112. MSF, May 3, 1893.
113. Mitchell, *Two Lives*, p. 110.
114. MSF, April 30, 1893.
115. MSF, May 23, 1893; June 3, 1893.
116. Rothman, *Living in the Shadow of Death*, p. 182.
117. Mitchell, *Two Lives*, p. 105.
118. MSF, Feb. 19, 1893.
119. Mitchell, *Two Lives*, pp.108–9.
120. MSF, Dec. 26, 1892.
121. MSF, Dec. 24, 1892.
122. Quoted in Antler, *Two Lives*, 14.
123. Antler, *Lucy Sprague Mitchell*, p. 36.
124. Mitchell, *Two Lives*, p. 111.
125. Mitchell, *Two Lives*, p. 37.
126. Mitchell, *Two Lives*, p. 125.
127. MSF, July 20, 1893.
128. Antler, *Lucy Sprague Mitchell*.
129. Jane Tompkins, *Sensational Designs: The Cultural Work of American Fiction, 1790–1860* (New York: Oxford University Press, 1985), p. 165.
130. MSF, May 30, 1893.
131. MLS.
132. See addenda to diaries, compiled by Cathryn Griffith.
133. MLS, Sept. 24, 1926.
134. MLS, Sept. 12, 1913.
135. Pottenger, *Fight against Tuberculosis*, p. 118.
136. Quoted in Rothman, *Living in the Shadow of Death*, pp. 196–97.
137. Godias J. Drolet, *Tuberculosis Hospitalization* (New York: New York Tuberculosis and Health Associaton, 1926), pp. 1–2.
138. Rothman, *Living in the Shadow of Death*, p. 220.
139. Rothman, *Living in the Shadow of Death*, p. 220.
140. MLS, "Another Last Night of Year, 1911."
141. Baur, *Health Seekers*, p. 60.
142. Pottenger, *Fight against Tuberculosis*, p. 88.
143. Pottenger, *Fight against Tuberculosis*, pp. 123–24.
144. MLS, Jan. 5, 1915.
145. *Land of Sunshine*, v. 1, no. 1 (June 1894), advertisements at end of issue.
146. Annual meeting of the Ladies and Hebrew Benevolent Society, 1902–1914, Series II, Minute Books, 1902–1977, JFSS. "Mrs. Rothstein" is a pseudonym.
147. Charles Dwight Willard to Sarah Hiestand, Dec. 23, 1910, CDW.
148. Charles Dwight Willard to Sarah Hiestand, Jan. 3, 1911, CDW.
149. George H. Kress and Walter Lindley, *A History of the Medical Profession of Southern California*, 2d ed. (Los Angeles: Press of the Times-Mirror Printing and Binding House, 1910), p. 179.
150. MLS, April 8, 1915.
151. Paul Groth, *Living Downtown: The History of Residential Hotels in the United States* (Berkeley: University of California Press, 1994), p. 92.
152. See Alice Kessler-Harris, *Out to Work: A History of Wage-Earning Women in the United States* (New York: Oxford University Press, 1982), pp. 124–25.
153. Susan M. Reverby, *Ordered to Care: The Dilemma of American Nursing, 1850–1945* (Cambridge, U.K.: Cambridge University Press, 1987), pp. 15–16.

154. MLS, July 6, 1913.

155. MLS, Sept. 2, 1913.

156. MLS, Sept. 14, 1914.

157. MLS, Sept. 18, 1914.

158. MLS, Oct. 25, 1914.

159. See Ellen D. Baer, "Nurses," in *Women, Health, and Medicine in America: A Historical Handbook*, ed. Rima D. Apple (New Brunswick, N.J.: Rutgers University Press, 1992), p. 454; Bates, *Bargaining for Life*, p. 200; Reverby, *Ordered to Care*, p. 95.

160. MLS, April 4, 1914.

161. MLS, Nov. 8, 1914.

162. MLS, July 13, 1913.

163. MLS, Sept. 30, 1913.

164. MLS, Sept. 6, 1913.

165. MLS, Dec. 31, 1913.

166. MLS, May 31, 1914.

167. MLS, Feb. 1, 1915; May 22, 1915.

168. MLS, Sept. 9, 1913.

169. MLS, Sept. 30, 1913.

170. MLS, Sept. 24, 1914.

171. MLS, Jan. 24,1915.

172. MLS, April 17, 1915.

173. MLS, Sept. 10,1913.

174. MLS, July 7, 1915.

175. MLS, Aug. 3, 1915.

176. MLS, July 21, 1915.

177. *A Directory of Sanatoria, Hospitals, Day Camps, and Preventoria for the Treatment of Tuberculosis in the United States* (New York: National Tuberculosis Association, 1923), p. 14.

178. MLS, addenda.

179. Cited in Jules Tygiel, "Metropolis in the Making: Los Angeles in the 1920s," in *Metropolis in the Making: Los Angeles in the 1920s*, ed. Tom Sitton and William Deverell (Berkeley: University of California Press, 2001), p. 2.

180. Clark Davis, "From Oasis to Metropolis: Southern California and the Changing Context of American Leisure," *Pacific Historical Review*, v. 61 (Aug. 1992): 367.

181. See Tygiel, "Metropolis in the Making," pp. 1–9

182. Davis, "Oasis to Metropolis," p. 362.

183. William Alexander McClung, *Landscapes of Desire: Anglo Mythologies of Los Angeles* (Berkeley: University of California Press, 2000), p. 23.

184. Davis, "Oasis to Metropolis," pp. 357–86; Tom Zimmerman, "Paradise Promoted."

185. Douglas Cazaux Sackman, *Orange Empire: California and the Fruits of Eden* (Berkeley: University of California Press, 2005), pp. 107–14.

Chapter 2   Strategies of Exclusion

1. See Nancy Tomes, *The Gospel of Germs: Men, Women, and the Microbe in American Life* (Cambridge, Mass.: Harvard University Press, 1998), pp. 114–27.

2. Deborah A. Stone, *The Disabled State* (Philadelphia: Temple University Press, 1984), p. 172.

3. *Nineteenth Biennial Report of the State Board of Health of California, for the Fiscal Years from July 1, 1904, to June 30, 1906* (Sacramento: State Printing Office, 1907), pp. 16–17.

4. *Twenty-first Biennial Report of the State Board of Health for the Fiscal Years from July 1, 1908, to June 30, 1910* (Sacramento: State Printing Office, 1911), p. 106.

5. *Twenty-second Biennial Report of the State Board of Health for the Fiscal Years from July 1, 1910, to June 30, 1912* (Sacramento: State Printing Office, 1913), p. 113.

6. Robert M. Fogelson, *The Fragmented Metropolis: Los Angeles, 1850–1930* (Cambridge, Mass.: Harvard University Press, 1967), p. 78.

7. *Twenty-fourth Biennial Report of the State Board of Health of California for the Fiscal Years from July 1, 1914, to June 30, 1916* (Sacramento: State Printing Office, 1917), p. 173.

8. "Board of Public Health Minutes," Dec. 4, 1915, California State Archives, Sacramento.

9. See Linda Bryder, "'Not Always One and the Same Thing': The Registration of Tuberculosis Deaths in Britain, 1900–1950," *Social History of Medicine*, v. 9, no. 2 (1996): 253–65. Indeed, statistics about all causes of mortality were notoriously inaccurate at the turn of the twentieth century. See Robert P. Hudson, review of Gerald Grob, "The Deadly Truth: A History of Disease in America," in *Bulletin of the History of Medicine*, v. 77, no. 4 (Winter 2003): 969.

10. Francis Marion Pottenger, *Fight against Tuberculosis: An Autobiography* (New York: Henry Schuman, 1952), p. 119.

11. See Elizabeth Fee and Evelynn M. Hammonds, "Science, Politics, and the Art of Persuasion: Promoting the New Scientific Medicine in New York City," in *Hives of Sickness: Public Health and Epidemics in New York City*, ed. David Rosner (New Brunswick, N.J.: Rutgers University Press, 1995), pp. 155–96; Paul Starr, *The Social Transformation of American Medicine: The Rise of a Sovereign Profession and the Making of a Vast Industry* (New York: Basic Books, 1982), p. 187.

12. See Bryder, "'Not Always One and the Same Thing.'"

13. *California State Board of Health Monthly Bulletin*, v. 2, no. 7 (Dec. 1906): 65.

14. See Howard Markel, *When Germs Travel: Six Major Epidemics That Have Invaded America and the Fears They Have Unleashed* (New York: Vintage Books, 2005), p. 32.

15. See, for example, George H. Kress, "Compulsory Registration and Fumigation in Pulmonary Tuberculosis, the Two Most Important of All Preventive Measures," *California State Board of Health Monthly Bulletin*, v. 2, no. 7 (Dec. 1906): 67.

16. Ernest A. Sweet, "Interstate Migration of Tuberculous Persons: Its Bearing on the Public Health, with Special Reference to the States of Texas and New Mexico," *Public Health Reports* (April 16, 1915): 1159.

17. See Sweet, "Interstate Migration," pp. 1156–57.

18. Sweet, "Interstate Migration," p. 1150.

19. "The Southern California Anti-Tuberculosis League," *Southern California Practitioner*, v. 21, no. 9 (Sept. 1906): 466–67. The author is identified only as a contributor to the journal.

20. See Gail Bederman, *Manliness and Civilization: A Cultural History of Gender and Race in the United States, 1880–1917* (Chicago: University of Chicago Press, 1995); Katherine Ott, *Fevered Lives: Tuberculosis in American Culture since 1870* (Cambridge, Mass.: Harvard University Press, 1996), pp. 13–14; Anthony E. Rotundo, *American Manhood: Transformations in Masculinity from the Revolution to the Modern Era* (New York: Basic Books, 1993).

21. Susan Sontag, *Illness as Metaphor* (New York: Vintage Books, 1979), pp. 11–12.

22. Petitions to the Board of Supervisors, August 20, 1908, file OD949H, LACBS.

23. See Barbara Gutmann Rosenkrantz, "Introductory Essay: Dubos and Tuberculosis, Master Teachers," in René and Jean Dubos, *Tuberculosis, Man, and Society* (New Brunswick, N.J.: Rutgers University Press, 1992), p. xxviii.

24. Hermann M. Biggs, *The Administrative Control of Tuberculosis* (New York: New York City Department of Health, 1909), p. 21.

25. Charles-Edward Armory Winslow, *The Life of Hermann Biggs, M.D., D.Sc., LL.D., Physician and Statesman of the Public Health* (Philadelphia: Lea & Febiger, 1929), p. 198.

26. New York City Charity Organization Society, *Home Treatment of Tuberculosis in New York City: Being a Report of the Relief Committee of the Committee on the Prevention of Tuberculosis of the New York City Charity Organization Society* (New York: New York City Charity Organization Society, 1908), p. 16.

27. See, e.g., Georgina D. Feldberg, *Disease and Class: Tuberculosis and the Shaping of Modern North American Society* (New Brunswick, N.J.: Rutgers University Press, 1956); Alan M. Kraut, *Silent Travelers: Germs, Genes, and the "Immigrant Menace"* (Baltimore: Johns Hopkins University Press, 1994); Markel, *When Genes Travel.*

28. Pottenger, *Fight against Tuberculosis*, p. 116.

29. Norman Bridge, "How Far Shall the State Restrict Individual Action of the Sick, Especially the Tuberculous," *California State Journal of Medicine*, v. 1 (1903): 180.

30. F. M. Pottenger, "Is Another Chapter in Public Phthisiophobia about to Be Written?" *California State Journal of Medicine*, Jan. 1903.

31. Pottenger, *Fight against Tuberculosis*, p. 116.

32. *California State Board of Health Monthly Bulletin*, v. 8, no. 7 (Jan. 1913): 124.

33. *Thirty-first Biennial Report of the Department of Public Health, July 1, 1928, to June 30, 1930* (Sacramento: State Printing Office, 1931).

34. William A. Sawyer, "Statement," *Hearings before the Committee on Public Health and National Quarantine*, U.S. Senate, 64th Congress, First Session on S. 202 (Washington, D.C.: Government Printing Office, 1916).

35. See Dr. Philip King Brown to Surgeon General Rupert Blue, Oct. 21, 1915; Philip King Brown to Assistant Secretary B. R. Newton, Oct. 23, 1915; Philip King Brown to Alexander Lambert, Oct. 19, 1915; W. A. Sawyer to Woodrow Wilson, Dec. 15, 1915; Philip King Brown to Rupert Blue, Nov. 30, 1915; W. A. Sawyer to Franklin K. Lane, Secretary of the Interior, Dec. 18, 1915; Norman Bridge to Wm. G. McAdoo, Secretary of the Treasury, Dec. 23, 1915 (all in file 5153, May–Dec. 1915, RG 90, Central File 1897–1923, Box 561, NACP).

36. See Edythe Tate-Thompson to Charles P. Hunt, Feb. 28, 1916, file 5153 (1916), RG 90, NACP.

37. "Board of Public Health Minutes," Jan.–March 1918, California State Archives, Sacramento.

38. Edythe Tate-Thompson to Hugh S. Cummings, Dec. 29, 1922, file 5153 (1922–23), RG 90, NACP.

39. *Twenty-eighth Biennial Report of the State Board of Health of California for the Fiscal Years from July 1, 1922, to June 30, 1924* (Sacramento: California State Printing Office, 1925), p. 63.

40. "The Problem of Poor Consumptives," *Southern California Practitioner* (April 1909): 212; see also JFSS.

41. Committee on the Prevention of Tuberculosis of the Charity Organization Society to "Dear Doctor," Nov. 27, 1905, reprinted in F. M. Pottenger, "Department of Tuberculosis," *Southern California Practitioner*, v. 21, no. 3 (March 1906): 128.

42. "Professional Beggar," *The Express*, Oct. 20, 1998.

43. *California State Board of Health Monthly Bulletin*, v. 1, no. 6 (Nov. 1905): 44.

44. Minute Books, 1902–1977, Series II, JFSS.

45. "The Problem of Poor Consumptives," *Southern California Practitioner*, v. 24, no. 4 (April 1909): 211.

46. P. M. Carrington, "Interstate Migration of Tuberculous Persons: Its Bearing on the Public Health with Reference to the State of California," *Public Health Reports* (March 19, 1915): 835–40.

47. *Annual Report of the Department of Health of the City of Los Angeles, California, for the Year Ended June 30, 1917* (Los Angeles: Department of Health, 1917), p. 33.

48. John E. Baur, *The Health Seekers of Southern California* (San Marino, Calif.: Huntington Library, 1959).

49. Los Angeles *Herald*, Nov. 11, 1902.

50. "Resolutions in Regard to Board of Supervisors and Proposed County Hospital," adopted Nov. 14, 1902, file OD 3110H, LACBS.

51. Los Angeles *Herald*, April 9, 1903.

52. See Benjamin Louis Cohen, "Constancy and Change in the Jewish Family Agency of Los Angeles: 1854–1970," Ph.D. dissertation, School of Social Work, University of Southern California, Los Angeles, June 1972, pp. 1–10; Max Vorspan and Lloyd P. Gartner, *History of the Jews of Los Angeles* (San Marino, Calif.: Huntington Library, 1970), p. 171.

53. *B'nai B'rith Messenger*, July 29, 1910.

54. Quoted in Vorspan and Gartner, *History of the Jews*, p. 109.

55. *B'nai B'rith Messenger*, Dec. 27, 1912.

56. See Jack Glazier, *Dispersing the Ghetto: The Relocation of Jewish Immigrants across America* (Ithaca, N.Y.: Cornell University Press, 1998).

57. Letter of Isaac Norton, *B'nai B'rith Messenger*, Feb. 14, 1913.

58. Maurice Salzman, "An Ounce of Prevention," *B'nai B'rith Messenger*, Oct. 13, 1911.

59. Vorspan and Gartner, *History of the Jews*, p. 173.

60. Letter of Isaac Norton, *B'nai B'rith Messenger*, March 14, 1913.

61. Letter of Isaac Norton, March 14, 1913.

62. Henry A. Strauss, "B'nai B'rith Lodge News," *B'nai B'rith Messenger*,, Feb. 14, 1913. On the controversy among Jewish tuberculosis organizations in Denver, see Jeanne Abrams, "Chasing the Cure in Colorado: The Jewish Consumptives' Relief Society," in *Jews of the American West*, ed. Moses Rischin and John Livingston (Detroit: Wayne State University Press, 1991), pp. 95–115.

63. Henry M. Silverberg, "History of the Jewish Consumptive Relief Association," in *Southwest Jewry: An Account of Jewish Progress and Achievement in the Southland*, ed. Joseph L. Malamut (Los Angeles: Sunland Publishing, 1926), p. 16.

Chapter 3   Creating a Tuburculosis Program

1. Experts now conclude that TB sanatoriums did indeed serve that purpose and that the decline of the disease probably stemmed from the spread of these institutions throughout the nation; see Howard Markel, *When Germs Travel: Six Major Epidemics That Have Invaded America and the Fears They Have Unleashed* (New York: Vintage Books, 2005), pp. 37–38.

2. Francis Marion Pottenger, *The Fight against Tuberculosis: An Autobiography* (New York: Henry Schuman, 1952), pp. 116–19.

3. Quoted in Helen Eastman Martin, *The History of the Los Angeles County Hospital and the Los Angeles County–University of Southern California Medical Center, 1968–1978* (Los Angeles: University of California Press, 1979), p. 37.

4. Martin, *Los Angeles County Hospital*, p. 37.

5. Figure 2-3 in Martin, *Los Angeles County Hospital*, p. 41.

6. Martin, *Los Angeles County Hospital*, p. 23.

7. Oct.17, 1914, file OD 1197, LACBS.

8. C.H.E. to Los Angeles County Board of Supervisors, Sept. 15, 1899, file OD 3085H, LACBS.

9. Martin, *Los Angeles County Hospital*, p. 43.

10. Quoted in Martin, *Los Angeles County Hospital*, p. 45.

11. George H. Kress and O. O. Witherbee, "The Los Angeles County Hospital," in *Southern California Practitioner*, v. 25, no. 6 (May 1910): 233–37.

12. "Over-crowded Conditions at County Hospital and Farm," Oct. 27, 1921, file OD 5088H, LACBS; C. H. Whitman, "A Few Remarks on the Los Angeles County Tuberculosis Problem," *Southern California Practitioner*, v. 27, no. 5 (May 1912): 207.

13. Edythe Tate-Thompson to L.A. County Board of Supervisors, Dec. 1921, file OD 5111H, LACBS.

14. See Martin, *Los Angeles County Hospital*, pp. 21–143.

15. *A Directory of Sanatoria, Hospitals, Day Camps, and Preventoria for the Treatment of Tuberculosis in the United States* (New York: National Tuberculosis Association, 1923), pp. 9–18.

16. Born in Ossining, New York, in 1868, Barlow attended Columbia University's College of Physicians and Surgeons and interned at Mount Sinai Hospital. Shortly after opening his medical practice, he received a tuberculosis diagnosis. Like many "wandering" poor, he moved frequently in search of a cure, traveling first to Denver and then to San Diego, before arriving in Los Angeles in 1897. As he gradually recovered, he began to treat many tuberculosis patients. Two years after founding his institution for the "indigent tuberculous of Los Angeles County," he established the Southern California Sanatorium for Nervous Disease for a more affluent clientele. See Robert Finegan, *The Barlow Story: An Illustrated History of Barlow Respiratory Hospital, 1902–1992* (Los Angeles: Barlow Respiratory Hospital, 1992), pp. 1–19; see also George H. Kress and Walter Lindley, *A History of the Medical Profession of Southern California* (Los Angeles: Times-Mirror Printing and Binding House, 1910), pp. 202–3.

17. Finegan, *Barlow Story*, p. 8.

18. R. L. Cunningham, "The Seventh Year at the Barlow Sanatorium, Los Angeles, Cal., Report on Sixty-Five Patients Discharged during the Year Sept. 1, 1909–Sept. 1, 1910," *Southern California Practitioner*, v. 26, no. 1 (Jan. 1911): 12.

19. Robert W. Poindexter, "Tuberculosis—A Layman's Idea," *Southern California Practitioner*, v. 20, no. 1 (Jan. 1905): 14.

20. W. Jarvis Barlow, "Report on Two Hundred Charity Cases of Pulmonary Tuberculosis, under Sanatorium Treatment at Los Angeles (1903–1907)," *Transactions of the American Climatological Association for the Year 1907*, v. 23 (1907): 163.

21. "The Third Annual Report of the Barlow Sanatorium for Poor Consumptives," *Southern California Practitioner*, v. 21, no. 11 (Nov. 1906): 579.

22. Barlow, "Report on Two Hundred Charity Cases," p. 162.

23. Finegan, *Barlow Story*, p. 22.

24. "Third Annual Report of Barlow Sanatorium," p. 579.

25. R. L. Cunningham, "The Barlow Sanatorium, Los Angeles, Cal. Report on Sixty-six Cases Discharged during the Year, September, 1908–September, 1909," *Southern California Practitioner*, v. 24, no. 12 (Dec. 1909): 607.

26. George H. Kress, "A Visit to the Barlow Sanatorium. A Los Angeles Institution for the Treatment of Pulmonary Tuberculosis," *Southern California Practitioner*, v. 20, no. 12 (Dec. 1905): 555–56.

27. "Twelfth Annual Report of La Viña, Pasadena, January 31, 1922," p. 17, HSC.

28. "Report of La Viña," p. 18.

29. Samuel H. Gotter, *The City of Hope* (New York: G. P. Putnam, 1954), p. xi; interview with Joseph Broady, City of Hope, Los Angeles, Oct. 21, 2002; Henry M. Silverberg, "History of the Jewish Consumptive Relief Association," in *Southwest Jewry: An Account of Jewish Progress and Achievement in the Southland*, ed. Joseph L. Malamut (Los Angeles: Sunland Publishing, 1926), p. 14.

30. Leon Shulman, "The California Consumptives' Relief Association," *The Sanatorium*, v. 7, no. 2 (March–April 1913): 39.

31. Paul Dembitzer, "Twenty Years," *Twentieth Anniversary: Los Angeles Sanatorium and Expatients Home* (Los Angeles: Jewish Consumptive and Expatients Relief Association, 1934), p. 44.

32. Silverberg, "History," p. 18.

33. *Thirty-first Biennial Report of the Department of Public Health, from July 1, 1928 to June 30, 1930* (Sacramento: State Printing Office, 1931), p. 133.

34. *Southern California Practitioner*, v. 20, no. 2 (Feb. 1905), pp. 71–72.

35. See A. B. Nye, "An Article to Think About," *California State Board of Health Monthly Bulletin*, v. 7, no. 6 (Dec. 1911): 153.

36. "Introductory," *Report of the California Tuberculosis Commission of the State Board of Health, Sacramento, California* (Sacramento: State Printing Office, 1914).

37. W. F. Snow, "California versus the Tubercle Bacillus," *California State Board of Health Monthly Bulletin*, v. 7, no. 6 (Dec. 1911): 147; "A Preliminary Abstract of the Final Report of the California Tuberculosis Commission," *California State Board of Health Monthly Bulletin*, v. 8, no. 7 (Jan. 1913): 147.

38. Snow, "California versus the Tubercle Bacillus," pp. 143–47.

39. *Twenty-second Biennial Report of the State Board of Health of California for the Fiscal Years from July 1, 1910, to June 30, 1912* (Sacramento: State Printing Office, 1913), p. 1.

40. See Testimony of Edith (sic) Tate-Thompson, Reporter's Transcript of Testimony, re: County Health Department, before Grand Jury of the Year 1936, LACBS; Francis Marion Pottenger, *The Fight against Tuberculosis: An Autobiography* (New York: Henry Schuman, 1952), p. 119.

41. Bogen was yet another physician who originally arrived in the West as a health seeker. Born in Sunbury, Pennsylvania, in 1874, he received his medical degree in 1896 and then practiced in a coal-mining town. After the outbreak of the Spanish American War two years later, he enlisted in the navy, where he remained until tuberculosis forced him to retire in 1909. For several years he traveled frequently in search of a cure, trying various places in Colorado, Arizona, Wyoming, and California. After his recovery he served as director of the Naval Hospital in San Diego and medical director of a Red Cross mission in Siberia before opening a private practice in Glendale. He was appointed Olive View superintendent in 1921. See Emil Bogen, *Surgeon Errant: The Life and Writings of William Henry Bucher, 1874–1934* (Los Angeles: The Angelus Press, 1935), pp. 1–8.

42. Bogen, *Surgeon Errant*, p. 122.

43. Georgina D. Feldberg, *Disease and Class: Tuberculosis and the Shaping of Modern North American Society* (New Brunswick, N.J.: Rutgers University Press, 1995), p. 102.

44. "Report of the Grand Jury Committee on Charities and Charitable Institutions," Nov. 12, 1925, file 40.20/49, LACBS.

45. Edythe Tate-Thompson to L.A. County Board of Supervisors, Aug. 5, 1920, file OD 141-0, LACBS.

46. Norman Martin to Board of Supervisors, Aug. 5, 1922, file OD 221-0, LACBS; W. H. Bucher to Board of Supervisors, Aug. 15, 1923, file OD 235-0, LACBS; see Robert Alan Bauman, "From Tuberculosis Sanatorium to Medical Center: The History of Olive View Medical Center, 1920–1989," M.A. thesis, University of California, Santa Barbara, April 1989, p. 33.

47. Bucher to Board of Supervisors, Aug. 15, 1923.

48. Matthew W. Roth, "Mulholland Highway and the Engineering Culture of Los Angeles in the 1920s," in *Metropolis in the Making: Los Angeles in the 1920s*, ed. Tom Sitton and William Deverell (Berkeley: University of California Press, 2001), p. 66.

49. W. H. Bucher to Board of Supervisors, Dec. 24, 1923, file OD 305-0, LACBS.

50. See Everett J. Gray to Board of Supervisors, June 19, 1936, file 40.20/283, LACBS.

51. H.G.T. to E.L.M. Thompson, April 30, 1921, file OD 174-0, LACBS.

52. Edythe Tate-Thompson to Board of Supervisors, May 25, 1918, file OD 15-0; Aug. 5, 1920, OD 141-0; Oct. 19, 1920, OD 149-0; Dec. 31, 1920, OD 163-0; Dec. 20, 1920, OD 155-0; Dec. 13, 1922, OD 230-0; June 27, 1924, OD 350-0, LACBS.

53. "18th Annual Report of Olive View Sanatorium, 1936–37," p. 3, file 40.20/337, LACBS.

54. Bauman, "Tuberculosis Sanatorium," p. 31; "18th Annual Report," p. 3.

55. Bauman, "Tuberculosis Sanatorium," p. 46.

56. Bauman, "Tuberculosis Sanatorium," pp. 42, 48; Bogen, *Surgeon Errant*, pp. 123–25.

57. See Thomas Dormandy, *The White Death: A History of Tuberculosis* (New York: New York University Press, 2000), pp. 249–63; Barron H. Lerner, *Contagion and Confinement: Controlling Tuberculosis along the Skid Road* (Baltimore: Johns Hopkins University Press, 1998), p. 62.

58. Bogen, *Surgeon Errant*, p. 127.

59. Bogen, *Surgeon Errant*, p. 124.

60. Bogen, *Surgeon Errant*, p. 133.

61. Bogen, *Surgeon Errant*, p. 130.

62. Bogen, *Surgeon Errant*, p. 130.

63. Bogen, *Surgeon Errant*, p. 131.

64. Bogen, *Surgeon Errant*, p. 122.

65. "Report of the Tuberculosis Service, Los Angeles County, Olive View Sanatorium, Olive View, California," in *Thirtieth Biennial Report of the Department of Public Health of California for the Fiscal Years from July 1, 1926, to June 30, 1928* (Sacramento: State Printing Office, 1929), p. 178.

66. See "Olive View Annual Report, 1935–36," HSC.

67. Quoted in Bauman, "Tuberculosis Sanatorium," p. 41.

68. Edythe Tate-Thompson to L.A. County Board of Supervisors, March 21, 1924, file OD 330-0, LACBS.

69. Edythe Tate-Thompson to L.A. County Board of Supervisors, April 24, 1929, file 40.20/111, LACBS.

70. W. H. Holland to L.A. County Board of Supervisors, May 2, 1929, file 40.20/111.

71. Lucy M. Rice to W. H. Holland, April 30, 1929, file 40.20/111.

72. *Southern California Practitioner*, v. 30, no. 5 (May 1915): 173.

73. George E. Malsbary, Secretary, Society for the Prevention of Tuberculosis, to "Gentlemen," Dec. 20, 1913, Council File 185, 1914, Los Angeles City Archives.

74. *Southern California Practitioner*, v. 30, no. 5 (May 1915): 173.

75. See *53,052 Lives: A Brief History of the Los Angeles Tuberculosis and Health Association with a Report of Activities for 1936* (Los Angeles: Los Angeles Tuberculosis and Health Association, 1936), no page numbers.

76. *Annual Report of Department of Health of the City of Los Angeles, California, for the Year Ended June 30, 1926* (Los Angeles: Department of Health, 1927), p. 39.

77. *Annual Report of Department of Health, City of Los Angeles, for the Year Ended June 30, 1928* (Los Angeles: Department of Health, 1928), p. 34.

78. See Ira V. Hiscock, "A Survey of Public Health Activities in Los Angeles County, California, for the Committee on Administrative Practice, American Public Health Association" (1928), file 180.3/114, LACBS; "Health Department of Los Angeles County, California, Annual Report Year Ended June 30, 1935," p. 7, file 180.3, LACBS.

79. See William Deverell, *Whitewashed Adobe: The Rise of Los Angeles and the Remaking of Its Mexican Past* (Berkeley: University of California Press, 2004), pp. 129–71.

80. See Matt Garcia, *A World of Its Own: Race, Labor and Citrus in the Making of Greater Los Angeles, 1900–1970* (Chapel Hill: University of North Carolina Press, 2001), pp. 64–79.

81. "Annual Report of County Health Officer to Board of Supervisors, Los Angeles County, for Calendar Year 1920," p. 21, file OD 1874.8H, LACBS.

82. "Annual Report of County Health Officer to Board of Supervisors, Los Angeles County, for Calendar Year 1923," p. 29, file OD 1874.8H, LACBS

83. Hisock, "Survey of Public Health Activities," part 2, p. 103.

84. Zdenka Buben to John L. Pomeroy, July 26, 1927, file 180.2/78, LACBS.

85. Everett W. Mattoon to L.A. County Board of Supervisors, Dec. 19, 1927, file 180.2/78.

86. Alfred F. Hess, "The Tuberculosis Preventorium," *The Survey*, v. 30 (Aug. 30, 1913): 666–68; Alfred F. Hess, "The Significance of Tuberculosis in Infants and Children," *Journal of the American Medical Association*, v. 72 (Jan. 11, 1919): 83–88.

87. Hess, "Tuberculosis Preventorium," p. 667.

88. Cynthia Anne Connolly, "Prevention through Detention: The Pediatric Tuberculosis Preventorium Movement in the United States, 1909–1951," Ph.D. dissertation in Nursing, University of Pennsylvania, 1999, p. 47.

89. Connolly, "Prevention through Detention," pp. 47–74.

90. See *53,052 Lives*.

91. See *Triennial Report of the Los Angeles Tuberculosis Association, 1924–1926* (Los Angeles: Los Angeles Tuberculosis Association, 1926), pp. 14–23.

92. E. Anthony Rotundo, *American Manhood: Transformations in Masculinity from the Revolution to the Modern Era* (New York: Basic Books, 1993), p. 258.

93. Mark Harrison and Michael Worboys, "A Disease of Civilisation," in *Migrants, Minorities, and Health: Historical and Contemporary Studies*, ed. Lara Marks and Michael Worboys (New York: Routledge, 1997), p. 96.

94. *1927 Report of the Los Angeles Tuberculosis Association* (Los Angeles: Los Angeles Tuberculosis Association, 1927), p. 11.

95. David Anthony Tyeeme Clark and Joane Nagel, "White Men, Red Masks: Appropriations of 'Indian' Manhood in Imagined Wests," in *Across the Great*

Divide: Cultures of Manhood in the American West, ed. Matthew Basso, Laura McCall, and Dee Garceau (New York: Routledge, 2001), pp. 109–30.

96. *1927 Report*, p. 12.

97. See Merlin Dwight Yoder, "Case Studies of Boys in the Los Angeles Tuberculosis and Health Association Preventorium," M.A. thesis, School of Social Work, University of Southern California, June 1936.

98. *Annual Report of Department of Health of the City of Los Angeles, California, for the Year Ended June 30, 1916* (Los Angeles: Department of Health, 1916), p. 18; *Annual Report of Department of Health of the City of Los Angeles, California, for the Year Ended June 30, 1928*, p. 48; The College Settlement, *The First Report of Instructive District Nursing, 1898–1907* (Los Angeles: College Settlement, 1907), pp. 8–9; The College Settlement, *The Fourteenth Report of Instructive District Nursing, 1911–1912* (Los Angeles: College Settlement, 1912), p. 10; Minutes of the Case Committee, JFSS.

99. *Annual Report of Department of Health of the City of Los Angeles, California, for the Year Ended June 30, 1917* (Los Angeles: Department of Health, 1917), p. 33.

100. *Annual Report of Department of Health of the City of Los Angeles, California, for the Year Ended June 30, 1919* (Los Angeles: Department of Health, 1919), p. 59.

101. *Annual Report of Department of Health of the City of Los Angeles, California, for the Year Ended June 30, 1915* (Los Angeles: Department of Health, 1915), p. 79; *First Report of Instructive District Nursing*, p. 9.

102. Emily K. Abel, "Taking the Cure to the Poor: Patients' Responses to New York City's Tuberculosis Program, 1894–1918," *American Journal of Public Health*, v. 87, no. 11 (Nov. 1997): 1808–15.

103. See *Report of Department of Health of City of Los Angeles for 1916*, p. 99; *Triennial Report of the Los Angeles Tuberculosis Association, 1924–1926*, p. 10, HSC.

104. See Frances Mae Reeves, "Housing Problems of the Tuberculous Clients in the Los Angeles County Central Welfare District: A Study in Administrative Procedure," M.A. thesis, School of Social Work, University of Southern California, Los Angles, June 1936, p. 35.

105. *Triennial Report of Los Angeles Tuberculosis Association*, p. 10.

106. See Reeves, "Housing Problems," p. 30.

107. Reeves, "Housing Problems," p. 49.

108. See Department of Charities, "Relief and Medical Service for the Indigent Sick and Dependent Poor of Los Angeles County, California: A Brief Statement of Some Features of the Problem" (1923), Haynes Collection, Box 145, folder 13, "L.A. County Hospital," Department of Special Collections, Charles E. Young Research Library, UCLA; *Annual Report of Department of Health of City of Los Angeles, California, for the Year Ended June 30, 1929*, p. 28.

109. F. A. Carmelia and F. W. Kratz, "Tuberculosis Control in Los Angeles City" (1940), p. 2, HSC; *Annual Report of Department of Health of the City of Los Angeles, California, for the Year Ended June 30, 1926* (Los Angeles: Health Department, 1926), p. 40.

110. *Annual Report of Department of Health of the City of Los Angeles, California, for the Year Ended June 30, 1918* (Los Angeles: Health Department, 1918), p. 35; *Annual Report of Department of Health of City of Los Angeles for the Year Ended June 30, 1919*, p. 46.

111. "Annual Report of County Health Officer for 1923," p. 83, file OD 1874.8H, LACBS.

112. Cited in Bauman, "Tuberculosis Sanatorium to Medical Center," p. 39.

113. Interview with Sakaye Shigekawa, M.D., Los Angeles, May 15, 2003; Minutes of Case Committee, Box 11, files 4, 13; Box 12, file 1, JFSS.

114. See R. L. Cunningham, "The Seventh Year at the Barlow Sanatorium," pp. 11–12.

115. Minutes of Case Committee, Box 12, file 15, JFSS. All patient names are pseudonyms. The first Jewish charities in Los Angeles were the Hebrew Benevolent Society and the Ladies Benevolent Society, both established in the nineteenth century. In 1916 they merged and in 1929 adopted the name of the Jewish Social Service Bureau. The name later was changed to the Jewish Family Service Society of Los Angeles.

116. Minutes of Case Committee, Box 12, file 12, JFSS.

117. W. F. Snow, "California versus the Tubercle Bacillus," *California State Board of Health Monthly Bulletin*, v. 7, no. 6 (Dec. 1911): 145.

118. Minutes of Case Committee, Box 11, file 14, JFSS.

119. See Mary E. Odem, *Delinquent Daughters: Protecting and Policing Adolescent Female Sexuality in the United States, 1880–1920* (Chapel Hill: University of North Carolina Press, 1995), p. 68.

120. See Minutes of Case Committee, Box 11, file 18, JFSS.

121. Max Vorspan and Lloyd P. Gartner, *History of the Jews of Los Angeles* (San Marino, Calif.: Huntington Library, 1970), pp. 176–77.

122. Minutes of Case Committee, JFSS.

123. Minutes of Case Committee, Box 12, file 12, JFSS.

124. National Tuberculosis Association, *A Directory of Sanatoria, Hospitals, Day Camps and Preventoria for the Treatment of Tuberculosis in the United States* (New York: National Tuberculosis Association, 1923), p. 16.

125. Becky M. Nicolaides, *My Blue Heaven: Life and Politics in the Working-Class Suburbs of Los Angeles, 1920–1965* (Chicago: University of Chicago Press, 2002), p. 72.

126. Interview with Mrs. Emilia Castañeda de Valenciana by Christine Valenciana, Sept. 8, 1971, OHP.

127. Mary Helen Ponce, *Hoyt Street: An Autobiography* (Albuquerque: University of New Mexico Press, 1993), p. 91.

128. Interview with Emilia Castañeda de Valenciana.

129. Carmelia and Kratz, "Tuberculosis Control in Los Angeles City," p. 16. Although Los Angeles contained an unusually high proportion of single-family homes, many newcomers rented accommodations at first. See Robert M. Fogelson, *The Fragmented Metropolis: Los Angeles, 1850–1930* (Cambridge, Mass.: Harvard University Press, 1967), p. 145.

130. Carmelia and Kratz, "Tuberculosis Control," p. 16.

131. Douglas Flamming, *Bound for Freedom: Black Los Angeles in Jim Crow America* (Berkeley: University of California Press, 2005), p. 306; Nicolaides, *My Blue Heaven*, p. 27; George Sánchez, *Becoming Mexican American: Ethnicity, Culture, and Identity in Chicano Los Angeles, 1900–1945* (New York: Oxford University Press, 1993), pp. 80–81.

132. Cited in Garcia, *A World of Its Own*, p. 96.

133. Cited in Camille Guerin-Gonzales, *Mexican Workers and American Dreams: Immigration, Repatriation, and California Farm Labor, 1900–1939* (New Brunswick, N.J.: Rutgers University Press, 1994), p. 67.

134. W. H. Holland to Board of Supervisors, Sept. 6, 1928, file 40.20/97, LACBS.

135. W. H. Holland to Board of Supervisors, April 10, 1931, file 40.20/133, LACBS.

136. Interview with Mrs. Antonia Monatones by Christine Valenciana, March 24, 1972, OHP.

137. Association of Tuberculosis Clinics and the Committee on the Prevention of Tuberculosis of the Charity Organization Society of the City of New York, *Tuberculosis Families in Their Homes: A Case Study* (New York: United Charities Building, 1916), p. 16.

138. Bureau of Public Health Education, "The Present Status of Anti-Tuberculosis Work," *Monthly Bulletin of the Department of Health of the City of New York*, v. 9 (Sept. 1916): 244.

139. See Simi Linton, *Claiming Disability: Knowledge and Identity* (New York: New York University Press, 1998); Rosemarie Garland Thomson, *Extraordinary Bodies: Figuring Physical Disability in American Culture and Literature* (New York: Columbia University Press, 1997).

140. Testimony of Tate-Thompson.

141. See Emily K. Abel, *Suffering in the Land of Sunshine: A Los Angeles Illness Narrative* (New Brunswick, N.J.: Rutgers University Press, 2006).

142. Cunningham, "Seventh Year of the Barlow Sanatorium," pp. 14–15.

143. "Report of Conference in Regard to Proposed Tubercular Clinics," Dec. 18, 1923, file OD 1821H, LACBS.

144. Nicolaides, *My Blue Heaven.*

145. Executive Secretary's Report, Los Angeles Tuberculosis and Health Association, Sept. 1933, GPC.

146. Minutes of Case Committee, Box 11, file 11, JFSS.

147. Minutes of Case Committee, Box 11, file 4, JFSS.

148. Deborah A. Stone, *The Disabled State* (Philadelphia: Temple University Press, 1984).

149. See Emily K. Abel, "Medicine and Morality: The Health Care Program of the New York Charity Organization Society," *Social Service Review*, v. 71, no. 4 (Dec. 1997): 634–51.

150. Paul K. Longmore, *Why I Burned My Book and Other Essays on Disability* (Philadelphia: Temple University Press, 2003), p. 76.

151. Cohen, "Constancy and Change," p. 10; "Investigation of Outdoor Relief of the Los Angeles County Charities Office," Jan. 8, 1915, p. 4, file OD 327-C, LACBS.

152. Oral history interview with Zdenka Buben, Social Welfare Archives, Doheny Library, University of Southern California.

153. See Joel F. Handler and Yeheskel Hasenfeld, *The Moral Construction of Poverty: Welfare Reform in America* (Newbury Park, Calif.: Sage Publications, 1991), p. 79.

154. "Investigation of Outdoor Relief," p. 1.

155. "Report of the Bureau of Tuberculosis," in the *Thirty-first Biennial Report of the Department of Public Health*, p. 134.

156. *1928 Report of the Los Angeles Tuberculosis Association* (Los Angeles: Los Angeles Tuberculosis Association, 1928), no page numbers.

157. Reeves, "Housing Problems"; "Report of the Bureau of Tuberculosis," in the *Thirty-first Biennial Report of the Department of Public Health*, p. 134.

158. "Report of the Bureau of Tuberculosis," in the *Thirty-first Biennial Report of the Department of Public Health*, pp. 134–35.

Chapter 4 "Outsiders"

1. See Laura Wexler, *Tender Violence: Domestic Visions in an Age of U.S. Imperialism* (Chapel Hill: University of North Carolina Press, 2002), pp. 30–31.

2. Quoted in Gail Bederman, *Manliness and Civilization: A Cultural History of Gender and Race in the United States, 1880–1917* (Chicago: University of Chicago Press, 1995), p. 134.

3. Bederman, *Manliness and Civilization*, pp. 1–44.

4. Charles Dwight Willard, "The Padres and the Indians," *Land of Sunshine*, v. 2, no. 4 (Sept. 1894): 10.

5. Harry Ellington Brook, *The Land of Sunshine, Southern California: An Authentic Description of Its Natural Features, Resources and Prospects, Containing Reliable Information for the Homeseeker, Tourist and Invalid* (Los Angeles: World's Fair Association and Bureau of Information, 1893), p. 11; see Nayan Shah, *Contagious Divides: Epidemics and Race in San Francisco's Chinatown* (Berkeley: University of California Press, 2001).

6. Brook, *Land of Sunshine*, p. 63.

7. Spencer G. Willard, "Why Southern California Is Prosperous," *Land of Sunshine*, v. 1, no. 3 (Aug. 1894): 60.

8. "Advertising the Orange Industry," *Land of Sunshine*, v. 2, no. 1 (Dec. 1894): 10.

9. "The Right Kind of People," *Land of Sunshine*, v. 2, no. 1 (Dec. 1894): 10.

10. Roger Daniels, *The Politics of Prejudice: The Anti-Japanese Movement in California and the Struggle for Japanese Exclusion* (Berkeley: University of California Press, 1962), p. 13.

11. See Edna Bonacich and John Modell, *The Economic Basis of Ethnic Solidarity: Small Business in the Japanese American Community* (Berkeley: University of California Press, 1980); Richard Steven Street, *Beasts of the Field: A Narrative History of California Farmworkers, 1769–1913* (Stanford, Calif.: Stanford University Press, 2004), pp. 497–526.

12. Quoted in Street, *Beasts of the Field*, p. 416.

13. Charles Dwight Willard, "Taking Stock for A.D. 1911," *California Outlook* (Jan. 6, 1912): 15–16.

14. Charles Dwight Willard to Sarah Hiestand, July 16, 1909, CDW.

15. See Leonard Dinnerstein and David M. Riemers, *Ethnic Americans: A History of Immigration*, 4th ed. (New York: Columbia University Press, 1999), p. 76.

16. See Alan M. Kraut, *Silent Travelers: Germs, Genes, and the "Immigrant Menace"* (New York: Basic Books, 1994).

17. "Annual Report of County Health Officer to Board of Supervisors, Los Angeles County, Los Angeles, for Calendar Year 1919," p. 24, LACBS.

18. "Annual Report of County Health Officer to Board of Supervisors, Los Angeles County, California, for Calendar Year 1921," p. 22, file OD 1689H, LACBS.

19. Judith Walzer Leavitt, *Typhoid Mary: Captive to the Public's Health* (Boston: Beacon Press, 1996).

20. Judith Walzer Leavitt, "'Typhoid Mary' Strikes Back: Bacteriological Theory and Practice in Early 20th-Century Public Health," in *Sickness and Health in America: Readings in the History of Medicine and Public Health*, 3d ed., Judith Walzer Leavitt and Ronald L. Numbers (Madison: University of Wisconsin Press, 1997), p. 557.

21. "Report of County Health Officer for Calendar Year 1921," p. 6.

22. Street, *Beasts of the Field*, p. 512.

23. See William Deverell, *Whitewashed Adobe: The Rise of Los Angeles and the Remaking of Its Mexican Past* (Berkeley: University of California Press, 2004), p. 26.

24. Deverell, *Whitewashed Adobe*, p. 26.

25. George J. Sánchez, *Becoming Mexican American: Ethnicity, Culture, and Identity in Chicano Los Angeles, 1900–1945* (New York: Oxford University Press, 1993), p. 19.

26. Sánchez, *Becoming Mexican American*, p. 13.

27. Deverell, *Whitewashed Adobe*, p. 11.

28. Charles D. Willard to May Willard, Feb. 27, 1886, CDW.
29. Joseph Phillis to Board of Education of Los Angeles County, Jan. 9, 1997, file OD 674H, LACBS.
30. *Municipal Affairs*, v. 2, no. 5 (May 1907):1–2; see also Sánchez, *Becoming Mexican American*, pp. 78–80.
31. See Bessie B. Stoddard, "The Courts of Sonoratown—The Housing Problem as It Is to Be Found in Los Angeles," *Charities and the Commons* (December 1905), reprinted in *Southern California Practitioner*, v. 21, no. 1 (Jan. 1906): 44.
32. Stoddard, "Courts of Sonoratown," p. 44.
33. Titian Coffey, "The Housing Conditions of Los Angeles," *Southern California Practitioner*, v. 21, no. 12 (Dec. 1906): 628.
34. *Municipal Affairs*, v. 1, no. 8 (August 1906): p. 3; see Reisler, Mark, "Always the Laborer, Never the Citizen: Anglo Perceptions of the Mexican Immigrant during the 1920s," *Pacific Historical Review*, v. 45 (May 1976): 231–54
35. David Sibley, *Geographies of Exclusion* (London and New York: Routledge, 1995), p. 56.
36. Coffey, "Housing Conditions," p. 624.
37. Coffey, "Housing Conditions," p. 624.
38. *Report of the Housing Commission of the City of Los Angeles, 1906–1908* (Los Angeles: The Commission, 1908), p. 12.
39. Coffey, "Housing Conditions," p. 628.
40. "Report of the Work of the Visiting Nurse for a Period of Sixty Days, County Health Department," file OD 1160, LACBS.
41. John L. Pomeroy to Board of Supervisors, June 29, 1916, file OD 1169, LACBS.
42. See Howard Markel, *When Germs Travel: Six Major Epidemics That Have Invaded America and the Fears They Have Unleashed* (New York: Vintage Books, 2005), pp. 111–40.
43. "First Annual Report of the Health Officer of Los Angeles County, California, for the Year Ending June 30, 1917," file OD 1260H, LACBS.
44. Amy L. Fairchild, *Science at the Borders: Immigrant Medical Inspection and the Shaping of the Modern Industrial Labor Force, 1891 to 1930* (Baltimore: Johns Hopkins University Press, 2003), p. 153; Markel, *When Germs Travel*, p. 134.
45. "Health Officer's Quarterly Report for December 31, 1916," file OD 1217H, LACBS.
46. Alfred W. Crosby, *America's Forgotten Pandemic: The Influenza of 1918* (Cambridge, U.K.: Cambridge University Press, 1989), p. xiv.
47. Pomeroy to Board of Supervisors, March 22, 1919, file OD 1448, LACBS.
48. Pomeroy to Board of Supervisors, Dec. 17, 1918, file OD1396H, LACBS.
49. William Deverell, "Plague in Los Angeles, 1924: Ethnicity and Typicality," in *Over the Edge: Remapping the American West*, ed. Valerie J. Matsumoto and Blake Allmendinger (Berkeley: University of California Press, 1999), p. 179.
50. Deverell, "Plague in Los Angeles," pp. 172–200.
51. See Kraut, *Silent Travelers*, pp. 78–96; Guenter Risse, "Epidemics and History: Ecological Perspectives and Social Responses," in *AIDS: The Burdens of History*, ed. Elizabeth Fee and Daniel Fox (Berkeley: University of California Press, 1988), pp. 33–66.
52. Deverell, "Plague in Los Angeles."
53. Gladys Patric, *A Study of the Housing and Social Conditions in the Ann Street District of Los Angeles, California* (Los Angeles, 1918).

54. "Annual Report of County Health Officer to Board of Supervisors, Los Angeles County, for Calendar Year 1919," p. 83.

55. "Annual Report of County Health Officer to Board of Supervisors for Calendar Year 1923," p. 83, file OD 1874.8H, LACBS.

56. California Bureau of Tuberculosis, *A Statistical Study of Sickness among the Mexicans in the Los Angeles County Hospital, from July 1, 1922, to June 30, 1925* (Sacramento: State Printing Office, 1925).

57. See *Annual Report of the Department of Health of the City of Los Angeles for the Year Ended June 30, 1917* (Los Angeles: Department of Health, 1917), p. 94; *Annual Report of the Department of Health of the City of Los Angeles for the Year Ended June 30, 1930* (Los Angeles: Department of Health, 1930), p. 331.

58. See Daniel J. Kevles, *In the Name of Eugenics: Genetics and the Uses of Human Heredity* (Cambridge, Mass.: Harvard University Press, 1985), p. 67.

59. See Allan M. Brandt, "Racism and Research: The Case of the Tuskegee Syphilis Study," *Hastings Center Report*, v. 8, no. 2 (1978): 21–29; B. W. Dippie, *The Vanishing American: White Attitudes and U.S. Indian Policy* (Middletown, Conn.: Wesleyan University Press, 1982); Katherine Ott, *Fevered Lives: Tuberculosis in American Culture since 1870* (Cambridge, Mass.: Harvard University Press, 1996), pp. 100–10; Marion M. Torchia, "Tuberculosis among American Negroes: Medical Research on a Racial Disease, 1830–1950," *Journal of the History of Medicine and Allied Sciences*, v. 32 (1977): 252–79; see also Douglas C. Baynton, "Disability and the Justification of Inequality in American History," in *The New Disability History, American Perspectives*, ed. Paul K. Longmore and Lauri Umansky (New York: New York University Press, 2001), pp. 33–57. On contemporary notions about racial susceptibility to disease among colonial populations, see Warwick Anderson, "Immunities of Empire: Race, Disease, and the New Tropical Medicine, 1900–1920," *Bulletin of the History of Medicine*, v. 70 (1996): 94–118, and Mark Harrison and Michael Worboys, "A Disease of Civilization: Tuberculosis in Britain, Africa, and India, 1900–1939," in *Migrants, Minorities and Health: Historical and Contemporary Studies*, ed. Lara Marks and Michael Worboys (London and New York: Routledge, 1997), pp. 93–124.

60. Ernest A. Sweet, "Interstate Migration of Tuberculous Persons: Its Bearing on the Public Health, with Special Reference to the States of Texas and New Mexico," *Public Health Reports*, v. 30, no. 17 (April 23, 1915): 1239. On contemporary notions about "civilization," see Bederman, *Manliness and Civilization*.

61. Sweet, "Interstate Migration," p. 1240.

62. On the racial formation of Mexicans, see Mae M. Ngai, *Impossible Subjects: Illegal Aliens and the Making of Modern America* (Princeton, N.J.: Princeton University Press, 2004).

63. Bederman, *Manliness and Civilization*, p. 193.

64. Nancy Tomes, *The Gospel of Germs: Men, Women, and the Microbe in American Life* (Cambridge, Mass.: Harvard University Press, 1998), p. 126.

65. Sheila M. Rothman, *Living in the Shadow of Death: Tuberculosis and the Social Experience of Illness in American History* (New York: Basic Books, 1994), pp. 183–85.

66. On school segregation, see Emory S. Bogardus, *The Mexican in the United States* (Los Angeles: University of Southern California Press, 1934); Martha Menchaca, *The Mexican Outsiders: A Community History of Marginalization and Discrimination in California* (Austin: University of Texas Press, 1995); Douglas Monroy, *Rebirth: Mexican Los Angeles from the Great Migration to the Great Depression* (Berkeley: University of California Press, 1999), pp. 132–37; Judith Rosenberg

Raftery, *Land of Fair Promise: Politics and Reform in Los Angeles Schools, 1885–1941* (Stanford, Calif.: Stanford University Press, 1992); Sánchez, *Becoming Mexican American.*

67. "Annual Report of County Health Officers to Board of Supervisors for Calendar Year 1923," p. 29.

68. Pomeroy to Board of Supervisors, June 8, 1925, file 180.2/9, LACBS.

69. Pomeroy to Board of Supervisors, April 11, 1927, file 180.2/66, LACBS.

70. "Annual Report of County Health Officer to Board of Supervisors for Calendar Year 1923," p. 30.

71. Pomeroy to Board of Supervisors, March 31, 1926, file 180.2/30, LACBS.

72. Pomeroy to Board of Supervisors, March 3, 1925, file 180.2/6+, LACBS; Pomeroy to Board of Supervisors, Aug. 21, 1928, file 180.3/112, LACBS.

73. Pomeroy to Board of Supervisors, March 3, 1925.

74. Pomeroy to Board of Supervisors, Aug. 21, 1928.

75. See Bogardus, *The Mexican,* p. 53; Raftery, *Land of Fair Promise*; Sánchez, *Becoming Mexican American,* p. 102.

76. Pomeroy to Board of Supervisors, Aug. 21, 1928.

77. Pomeroy to Board of Supervisors, March 3, 1925.

78. Pomeroy to Board of Supervisors, June 6, 1923, OD 1754H, LACBS.

79. Pomeroy to Board of Supervisors, Aug. 21, 1928; "Annual Report of the Los Angeles County Department of Health for 1929–30," p. 43, file 180.3/172, LACBS.

80. *Twenty-eighth Biennial Report of the State Board of Health of California for the Fiscal Years from July 1, 1922, to June 30, 1924* (Sacramento: State Printing Office, 1925), p. 65.

81. Notes attached to letter from Sidney M. Maguire to George P. Clements, September 29, 1928, Box 62, GPC.

82. *Triennial Report of the Los Angeles Tuberculosis Association, 1924–1926* (Los Angeles: Los Angeles Tuberculosis Association, 1927), p. 14.

83. Violet Blanche Goldberg, "A Study of the Home Treatment of Tuberculosis Cases with Details of a Colony Plan in Los Angeles County and a Study of a Family Group of Ninety-Nine," M.A. thesis, University of Southern California School of Social Work, Los Angeles, June 1939, p. 7.

84. Benjamin Goldberg, "Tuberculosis in Racial Types with Special Reference to Mexicans," *American Journal of Public Health,* v. 19 (March 1929): 281.

85. Mrs. H.K.M. Bent to Los Angeles County Board of Supervisors, Feb. 9, 1916, file OD 1283-C, LACBS.

86. Interview of Emilia Castañeda de Valenciana by Christine Valenciana, Sept. 8, 1971, OHP.

87. Quoted in Sánchez, *Becoming Mexican American,* p. 99.

88. Sidney M. Maguire, Executive Secretary, to Officers and Members of the Los Angeles Tuberculosis Association, Jan. 1921, HSC; see Emil Bogen, *Surgeon Errant: The Life and Writings of William Henry Bucher, 1874–1934* (Los Angeles: The Angelus Press, 1935), p. 134.

89. John L. Pomeroy to Board of Supervisors, March 15, 1916, file OC 1140H, LACBS; Pomeroy to Board of Supervisors, March 27, 1916, file OD1145H, LACBS.

90. "Annual Report of County Health Officer to Board of Supervisors, Los Angeles County, California, for Calendar Year 1920," pp. 30, 40–44, OD 1874.8H.

91. Sánchez, *Becoming Mexican American,* p. 100.

92. "Annual Report for Calendar Year 1920," p. 42.

93. A physician at a city tuberculosis clinic wrote in 1917: "I am of the opinion that a great deal of unnecessary time is wasted in taking the history of the foreign population, which, as you know, is large in this city, because I discovered on careful reading and investigation that none of the histories with a few exceptions, were dependable. . . . Where the patients were intelligent American people, the history was of value. Where they were of Jewish extraction [or] of Spanish extraction, I found that the history was of little value." See *Annual Report of Department of Health of the City of Los Angeles, California, for the Year Ended June 30, 1917*, p. 32. In 1934, a social work student explained the need to substitute out-patient services for placement at Olive View this way: "The average Mexican patient . . . is uneasy in a strange setting, where the staff is of another race and speaks a language unfamiliar to most of the older Mexicans." See Goldberg, "A Study of the Home Treatment," p. 9.

94. Manuel Gamio, *The Life Story of the Mexican Immigrant: Autobiographic Documents* (New York: Dover Publications, 1971), p. 52.

95. *Statistical Study.*

96. *Statistical Study.*

97. *Summary of Mexican Cases Where Tuberculosis Is a Problem* (Sacramento: State Printing Office, 1926).

98. See Mae M. Ngai, "The Architecture of Race in American Immigration Law: A Reexamination of the Immigration Act of 1924," *Journal of American History*, v. 86, no. 1 (June 1999).

99. Ngai, "Illegal Aliens and Alien Citizens."

100. Mae Ngai, "The Strange Career of the Illegal Alien: Immigration Restriction and Deportation Policy in the United States, 1921–1965," *Law and History Review*, v. 21, no.1 (Spring 2003): 69–108.

101. *Statistical Study.*

102. TMR, Sept. 17, 1934.

103. *Grizzly Bear*, Dec. 1927.

104. Fairchild, *Science at the Borders.*

105. On employers' attitudes, see Aristide R. Zolberg, *A Nation by Design: Immigration Policy in the Fashioning of America* (Cambridge, Mass.: Harvard University Press, 2006), pp. 254–58.

106. "Department of Health, Los Angeles County, Quarterly Report for December 31, 1916," file OD1217H, LACBS.

107. *Mexicans in California: Report of Governor C. C. Young's Mexican Fact-Finding Committee* (San Francisco, Oct. 1930), p. 187.

108. Edythe Tate-Thompson, "Public Health among the Mexicans," paper read at the Annual Conference of the Friends of Mexico, Pomona College, Nov. 17, 1928, HR 71A-F16.4, NAW.

109. Edythe Tate-Thompson to Albert Johnson, Jan. 17, 1928, HR 70A-F14.3, NAW.

110. Tate-Thompson to Johnson, Feb. 1, 1930, HR 71A-F16.2, NAW.

111. Tate-Thompson to Johnson, Feb. 18, 1930, HR 71A-F16.2, NAW.

112. Emory S. Bogardus, *The Mexican in Los Angeles* (Los Angeles: University of Southern California Press, 1934), p. 84.

113. Petition, June 4, 1928, RG 233, Committee Papers, HR 70A-F14.3, NAW.

114. A. S. Baker to Albert Johnson, Jan. 30, 1928, HR 70A-F14.13, NAW.

115. *Western Hemisphere Immigration*, Hearings before the Committee on Immigration and Naturalization, House of Representatives, 71st Congress, Second Session on the Bills HR 8523, HR 8530, HR 8702, to Limit the Immigration of Aliens to the United States, and for Other Purposes (Washington, D.C.: Government Printing Office), p. 407.

116. *Immigration from Counties of the Western Hemisphere*, Hearings before the Committee on Immigration and Naturalization, House of Representatives, 70th Congress, First Session on HR 6465, HR 7358, HR 10955, HR 1168, Feb. 21, to April 5, 1928, Hearing No. 70.1.5 (Washington, D.C.: Government Printing Office, 1928), pp. 52, 59, 64, 90; *Seasonal Agricultural Laborers from Mexico*, Hearings before the Committee on Immigration and Naturalization, House of Representatives, 69th Congress, First Session, Jan. 28 and 29, Feb. 2, 9, 11, and 23, 1926, on HR 6741, HR 7559, HR 9036, Hearing No. 69.1.7 (Washington, D.C.: Government Printing Office, 1926), pp. 15, 319.

117. See Nayan Shah, *Contagious Divides: Epidemics and Race in San Francisco's Chinatown* (Berkeley: University of California Press, 2001).

118. Emil Bogen, "Racial Susceptibility to Tuberculosis," *American Review of Tuberculosis*, v. 24, no. 4 (1931): 522–31; quotation on p. 523.

119. Bogen, "Racial Susceptibility," p. 526.

Chapter 5   Slashing Services in the Great Depression

1. Richard David Lester, "Building the New Deal State on the Local Level: Unemployment Relief in Los Angeles County during the 1930s," Ph.D. dissertation, University of California, Los Angeles, 2001, pp. 57–58; see William H. Mullins, *The Depression and the Urban West, 1929–1933: Los Angeles, San Francisco, Seattle, and Portland* (Bloomington: Indiana University Press, 1991), pp. 14–72.

2. See Clark Davis, "From Oasis to Metropolis: Southern California and the Changing Context of American Leisure," *Pacific Historical Review*, v. 61 (Aug. 1992): 368.

3. Don Thomas to Harry Chandler, Nov. 9, 1939, Box 23, GLAVCB.

4. Addison B. Day to John R. Quinn, no date, file: Correspondence, L.A. County, Box 23, GLAVCB.

5. Minutes of Management Committee, April 4, 1934, GLAVCB.

6. Quoted in Tom Zimmerman, "Paradise Promoted: Boosterism and the L.A. Chamber of Commerce," *California History*, v. 64 (Winter 1985): 33; see also Davis, "From Oasis to Metropolis," p. 368.

7. TMR, Jan. 1939.

8. Minutes of Management Committee, Oct. 26, 1939, GLAVCB.

9. "Appropriations of Los Angeles County to the All-Year Club of Southern California," Box 25, GLAVCB.

10. TMR, Sept. 7, 1933.

11. "Annual Report of the Board of Health Commissioners, City of Los Angeles, California, for the Fiscal Year Ended June 30, 1936," p. 7, HSC.

12. "Annual Report of the Department of Health, City of Los Angeles, 1930–31,"no page number, HSC.

13. "Annual Report of Board of Health Commissioners, City of Los Angeles, for Year Ended June 30, 1936," p. 23, HSC.

14. "Annual Report of the Board of Health Commissioners, City of Los Angeles, Fiscal Year 1938–1939," p. 17, HSC.

15. See M. H. Lewis, *Transients in California: Special Surveys and Studies* (San Francisco: State Relief Administration of California, 1936), p. 5.

16. California's rate, however, was much lower than that in other states. In 1939 Thompson wrote that Michigan was "now paying $10 a week, Wisconsin $7, and a number of states $5" (TMR, Jan. 1939).

17. "18th Annual Report of Olive View Sanatorium, 1936–37," p. 19, file 40.20/337, LACBS.

18. Alberta Gude Lynch, President, Business Women's Legislative Council of California, to Board of Supervisors, June 27, 1934, file 40.20/338.1, LACBS.

19. TMR, Sept. 1936.

20. TMR, Aug. 1933.

21. Interview with Emilia Castañeda de Valenciana by Christine Valenciana, Sept. 8, 1971, OHP.

22. TMR, Jan. 1933.

23. TMR, Feb. 1933.

24. TMR, Oct. 1933.

25. "18th Annual Report of Olive View Sanatorium, 1936–37," p. 72.

26. TMR, June 1934.

27. Everett J. Gray to Board of Supervisors, April 28, 1936, file 40.20/274, LACBS.

28. TMR, Nov. 1940.

29. H. F. Scoville to Board of Supervisors, Aug. 23, 1938, file 40.20/338.1, LACBS.

30. Helen Eastman Martin, *The History of the Los Angeles County Hospital and the Los Angeles County–University of Southern California Medical Center, 1968–1978* (Los Angeles: University of California Press, 1979), p. 118.

31. TMR, Sept. 1934.

32. TMR, Jan. 1935.

33. TMR, Jan. 1935.

34. Quoted in Paul Starr, *The Social Transformation of American Medicine: The Rise of a Sovereign Profession and the Making of a Vast Industry* (New York: Basic Books, 1982), p. 182. See Charles E. Rosenberg, "Social Class and Medical Care in Nineteenth-Century America: The Rise and Fall of the Dispensary," *Journal of the History of Medicine and Allied Sciences*, v. 29 (1974): 32–54.

35. See John L. Pomeroy, "Administration of Public Health: Viewpoints of Public Health Experts and Los Angeles County Medical Society," file 180.3/254, LACBS.

36. See George H. Kress to John L. Pomeroy, April 5, 1932, file 180.2/212.5, LACBS.

37. John L. Pomeroy to Supervisor Henry W. Wright, June 19, 1931, file 180.2/212.1, LACBS.

38. Everett W. Mattoon to Los Angeles County Board of Supervisors, July 27, 1931, file 180.2/212.2, LACBS.

39. Pomeroy to Board of Supervisors, Feb. 10, 1932, file 180.2/212.5, LACBS.

40. See Pomeroy, "Administration of Public Health."

41. John L. Pomeroy to Board of Supervisors, Aug. 29, 1933, file 180.3/254, LACBS.

42. Zdenka Buben to John L. Pomeroy, Oct. 9, 1933, in Pomeroy, "Administration of Public Health," p. 86.

43. Kendall Emerson to Pomeroy, Sept. 16, 1933, in Pomeroy, "Administration of Public Health," pp. 15–16.

44. Haven Emerson to Pomeroy, Sept. 19, 1933, in Pomeroy, "Administration of Public Health," pp. 32–33.

45. Graham A. Laing to Pomeroy, Sept. 24, 1933, in Pomeroy, "Administration of Public Health," p. 39.

46. John P. Koehler to Pomeroy, Sept. 11, 1933, in Pomeroy, "Administration of Public Health," pp. 51–52.

47. See Paul K. Longmore *Why I Burned My Book and Other Essays* (Philadelphia: Temple University Press, 2003), pp. 53–101.

48. Interview with Frances Feldman, University of Southern California, Los Angeles, Dec. 6, 2002.

49. Edward J. Hanna, *Report and Recommendations of the California State Unemployment Commission* (Sacramento: State Printing Office, 1933), p. 371.
50. Hanna, *Unemployment Commission*, p. 337.
51. Hanna, *Unemployment Commission*, p. 348; Helen R. Jeter, *The Administration of Funds for Unemployment Relief by the Los Angeles County Department of Charities, prior to November 24, 1933, a Report Submitted to the Sub-Committee on Relief Standards and Procedure of the Los Angeles County Emergency Relief Committee* (Los Angeles: Los Angeles County Emergency Relief Committee, 1933), pp. 21–22; Lester, "Building the New Deal State," p. 70. Jeter noted that relief expenditures in Los Angeles County "during the second half of the fiscal year 1931–32 were below expenditures in Pittsburgh, Buffalo, Detroit, Philadelphia, and Boston."
52. Frances Mae Reeves, "Housing Problems of the Tuberculous Clients in the Los Angeles County Central Welfare District, A Study in Administrative Procedure," M.A. thesis, School of Social Work, University of Southern California, June 1936, pp. 36–40, LACBS
53. Harry Cohn to Board of Supervisors, July 7, 1931, file 40.31/393, LACBS.
54. TMR, May 1934.
55. "Report of the Committee on Tuberculosis Appointed by Mr. Earl E. Jensen, Superintendent of Charities," included in TMR, Aug. 1934.
56. TMR, April 1934.
57. "Report of Committee of Nutritionists Regarding the Adequacy of County Indigent Budget," Aug. 19, 1938, Box 64, file B III 14 c bb aaa, JAF.
58. W. R. Harriman to John Anson Ford, Sept. 16, 1938, Box 64, file B III 14 c bb aaa, JAF.
59. TMR, Dec. 1938.

Chapter 6   Expelling Mexicans and Filipinos

1. Mary Helen Ponce, *Hoyt Street: An Autobiography* (Albuquerque: University of New Mexico Press, 1993), p. 97.
2. Ponce, *Hoyt Street*, p. 9.
3. *Mexicans in California: Report of Governor C. C. Young's Mexican Fact-Finding Committee*, San Francisco, Oct. 1930, p. 194.
4. "Annual Report of the Los Angeles County Health Department for 1936–37," p. 7, file 180.3, LACBS.
5. "Annual Report of the Los Angeles County Health Department for 1937–38," p. 18, file 180.3, LACBS.
6. See Edward J. Escobar, *Race, Police, and the Making of a Political Identity: Mexican Americans and the Los Angeles Police Department, 1900–1945* (Berkeley: University of California Press, 1999), p. 122.
7. Ponce, *Hoyt Street*, p. 228.
8. "Annual Report of the Los Angeles County Health Department for 1937–38," p. 21.
9. Emil Bogen, "Racial Susceptibility to Tuberculosis, *American Review of Tuberculosis*, v. 24, no. 4 (1931): 523.
10. "Annual Report of the Los Angeles County Health Department for 1937–38," p. 10.
11. "Annual Report of the Los Angeles County Health Department for 1937–38," p. 12.
12. Nancy Tomes, *The Gospel of Germs: Men, Women, and the Microbe in American Life* (Cambridge, Mass.: Harvard University Press, 1998), p. 126.
13. "Annual Report of the Los Angeles County Health Department for 1937–38," p. 12.
14. "Annual Report of the Los Angeles County Health Department for 1937–38," p. 11.
15. "Annual Report of the Los Angeles County Health Department for 1937–38," p. 11.

16. "Annual Report of the Los Angeles County Health Department for 1937–38," p. 18.

17. "February [1938] Report of Department of Charities, Los Angeles County," p. 5, Box 64, file B14 c bb aaa, JAF.

18. TMR, July 1934.

19. TMR, April 1933.

20. TMR, July 1934.

21. TMR, March 1925.

22. TMR, Jan. 1933.

23. TMR, Jan. 1933.

24. "Fernandez" is a pseudonym.

25. TMR, Jan. 1933.

26. TMR, Oct. 1933.

27. TMR, May 1933.

28. TMR, Oct. 1933.

29. TMR, Jan. 1934.

30. TMR, Dec. 1937.

31. "Tuberculosis Control in Los Angeles City, from the Report by Medical Director F. A. Carmelia and P.A. Surgeon F. W. Kratz, U.S. Public Health Service, May 1940," p. 12, University of California Southern Regional Library Facility.

32. Letter from W. F. French to Rex Thomson, April 24, 1934, file 55853, Record Group 85, NAW.

33. W. H. Holland to J. H. Bean, February 4, 1927, file 40.20/75, LACBS; "17th Annual Report of Olive View Sanatorium, 1935–36," file 40.20, LACBS.

34. "Report of the Tuberculosis Colony in Huntington Park for the Year Ending 1933," file 180.3/264/40.31, LACBS.

35. Violet Blanche Goldberg, "A Study of the Home Treatment of Tuberculosis Cases with the Details of a Colony Plan in Los Angeles County and a Study of a Family Group of Ninety-Nine," M.A. thesis, School of Social Work, University of Southern California, 1939, p. 7.

36. "Report of the Tuberculosis Colony."

37. TMR, June 1935.

38. Edythe Tate-Thompson, "Report of the Bureau of Tuberculosis, July 1, 1928, to June 30, 1930," in *Thirty-first Biennial Report of the Department of Public Health of California for the Fiscal Years from July 1, 1928, to June 30, 1930* (Sacramento: State Printing Office, 1930), p. 174.

39. Herbert I. Sauer, "The Permanence of Rehabilitation Efforts: A Study of Rehabilitation of the Tuberculous in Los Angeles County, March 29, 1941," p. 10, University of California Southern Regional Library Facility.

40. Everett W. Mattoon to John L. Pomeroy, Jan. 30, 1932, file 180.3/254, LACBS.

41. "Annual Report of the Los Angeles County Health Department for 1939–40," p. 38, file 180.3/490, LACBS.

42. TMR, June 1932.

43. "Annual Report of the Los Angeles County Health Department for 1937–38," p. 11.

44. "Annual Report of the Los Angeles County Health Department for 1937–38," p. 63.

45. "Annual Report of the Los Angeles County Health Department for 1937–38," p. 63.

46. *Mexicans in California*, p. 187.

47. See George Sánchez, *Becoming Mexican American: Ethnicity, Culture, and Identity in Chicano Los Angeles, 1900–1945* (New York: Oxford University Press, 1993), pp. 211–12.

48. See Latin-American Protective League, "Resolution," 1933, file 40.31/821, LACBS.

49. Address of Earl Jensen, Patriotic Hall, Aug. 28, 1933, Box 64, file B 14 c bb aaa, JAF.

50. Latin-American Protective League, "Resolution."

51. Mabel Weed and Miss Eldridge, "Investigation of Outdoor Relief of the Los Angeles County Charities Office," 1915, file OD 327C, LACBS.

52. See Barbara J. Nelson, "The Origins of the Two-Channel Welfare State: Workmen's Compensation and Mothers' Aid," in *Women, the State, and Welfare*, ed. Linda Gordon (Madison: University of Wisconsin Press, 1990), pp. 123–51.

53. United Council of Working Class Women to Los Angeles County Board of Supervisors, October 29, 1934, file 40.31/1184, LACBS. An investigation by the Department of Charities concluded that the director "did err in summoning the policy" but also noted that the council shared an office with the Communist Party (W. G. Golden to Murray Moran, Nov. 8, 1934, file 40.31/1184, LACBS).

54. See especially Francisco E. Balderrama and Raymond Rodríguez, *Decade of Betrayal: Mexican Repatriation in the 1930s* (Albuquerque: University of New Mexico Press, 1995); Abraham Hoffman, *Unwanted Mexican Americans in the Great Depression: Repatriation Pressures, 1929–1939* (Tucson: University of Arizona Press, 1974); Sánchez, *Becoming Mexican American*.

55. Cited in Sánchez, *Becoming Mexican American*, p. 214.

56. Cited in Hoffman, *Unwanted Mexican Americans*, p. 44.

57. W. F. Watkins to Robe Carl White, Los Angeles, Feb. 21, 1931, file 55739/674, RG85, NAW.

58. Watkins to White, Feb. 21, 1931.

59. Hoffman, *Unwanted Mexican Americans*, pp. 59–60.

60. Reuben Oppenheimer, *The Administration of the Deportation Laws of the United States*, a report to the National Commission on Law Observance and Enforcement, 1931, p. 35.

61. Carrie Belle H. MacCarthy, "A Survey of the Mexican Hardship Cases Active in the Los Angeles County Department of Charities, Los Angeles, California," M.A. thesis, School of Social Work, University of Southern California, June 1939, p. 66.

62. Sánchez, *Becoming Mexican American*, p. 41.

63. Mai Ngai, "The Strange Career of the Illegal Alien: Immigration Restriction and Deportation Policy in the United States, 1921–1965," *Law and History Review*, v. 21, no. 1 (Spring 2003): 69–108.

64. Edythe Tate-Thompson, "Report of the Bureau of Tuberculosis," in *Thirty-first Biennial Report of the Department of Public Health of California for the Fiscal Years from July 1, 1928, to June 30, 1930*, p. 128.

65. *Thirty-second Biennial Report of the Department of Public Health of California for the Fiscal Years from July 1, 1930 to June 30, 1932* (Sacramento: State Printing Office, 1932), p. 132.

66. TMR, Oct. 1933.

67. MacCarthy, "Survey," p. 83.

68. TMR, May 2, 1934.

69. W. F. Watkins to Robe Carl White, Los Angeles, Feb. 8, 1931, and Feb. 21, 1931, file 5738/674, RG 85, NAW.

70. Los Angeles Tuberculosis and Health Association, Executive Secretary's Report, April 1934, GPC.

71. Interview with Frances Feldman, University of Southern California, Los Angeles, Dec. 6, 2002.

72. See Oppenheimer, *Administration*, pp. 31, 100.

73. As several historians note, the term "repatriation" is a misnomer because many people who were "returned" to Mexico had been born in the United States.

74. Balderrama and Rodríguez, *Decade of Betrayal*, p. 99; Camille Guerin-Gonzales, *Mexican Workers and American Dreams: Immigration, Repatriation, and California Farm Labor, 1900–1930* (New Brunswick, N. J.: Rutgers University Press, 1994), p. 84; Hoffman, *Unwanted Mexican Americans*, p. 91.

75. Hoffman, *Unwanted Mexican Americans*, p. 87.

76. J. H. Winslow to Rex Thomson, Los Angeles, Jan. 26, 1934, file 55853/737, RG 85, NAW.

77. MacCarthy, "Survey," p. 57.

78. Interview of Emilia Castañeda de Valenciana by Christine Valenciana, Sept. 8, 1971, OHP.

79. Rex Thomson to Alejandro V. Martinez, Los Angeles, Jan. 29, 1934, file 55853/737, RG 85, NAW.

80. Rex Thomson to Los Angeles County Board of Supervisors, Los Angeles, Feb. 15, 1934, file 40.31/340.35, LACBS.

81. Rex Thomson to Los Angeles County Board of Supervisors, Los Angeles, March 21, 1935, file 40.31/340.46, LACBS.

82. Winifred Ryle to A. C. Price, Los Angeles, Aug. 1, 1930, file 40.31/297, LACBS.

83. A. C. Price to Board of Supervisors, Los Angeles, July 20, 1938, file 40.31/858 LACBS.

84. See Rex Thomson to Los Angeles County Board of Supervisors, Sept. 30, 1935, file 40.31/1366, LACBS; Thomson to Board of Supervisors, Oct. 7, 1935, file 40.31/1386, LACBS; Thomson to Board of Supervisors, March 25, 1936, file 40.31/1425, LACBS.

85. TMR, March 31, 1934.

86. Sánchez, *Becoming Mexican American*, pp. 209–26.

87. Goldberg, "A Study of the Home Treatment of Tuberculosis Cases," p. 47.

88. Rex Thomson to Los Angeles County Board of Supervisors, May 25, 1937, file 40.31/340.47, LACBS.

89. Thomson to Board of Supervisors, May 25, 1937.

90. Thomson noted, however, that the figures he provided were only approximations.

91. Thomson to Board of Supervisors, May 25, 1937.

92. Rex Thomson to Los Angeles County Board of Supervisors, February 10, 1938, May 16, 1938, Aug. 9, 1938, Oct. 18, 1938, file 40.43/340, LACBS.

93. Hoffman, *Unwanted Mexican Americans*, p. 159.

94. File 40.31/340, LACBS.

95. Gordon L. McDonough to Los Angeles County Board of Supervisors, Nov. 21, 1938, file 40.31/340, LACBS.

96. McDonough to Board of Supervisors, Nov. 21, 1938.

97. McDonough to Board of Supervisors, Nov. 21, 1938.

98. McDonough to Board of Supervisors, Nov. 21, 1938.

99. McDonough to Board of Supervisors, Nov. 21, 1938.

100. See Balderrama and Rodríguez, *Decade of Betrayal*, p. 90.

101. L. E. Lampton to J. H. O'Connor, Dec. 6, 1938, file 30.41/340, LACBS.

102. See Balderrama and Rodríguez, *Decade of Betrayal*, p. 90.

103. Lampton to O'Connor, Dec. 6, 1938.

104. Sánchez, *Becoming Mexican American*, p. 210.

105. *Thirty-second Biennial Report of the Department of Public Health*, p. 132.

106. See Escobar, *Race, Police, and the Making of a Political Identity*, pp. 150–54; David Gutiérrez, *Walls and Mirrors: Mexican Americans, Mexican Immigrants, and the*

Politics of Identity (Berkeley: University of California Press, 1995), pp. 110–16; Vicki Ruiz, *From Out of the Shadows: Mexican Women in Twentieth-Century America* (New York: Oxford University Press, 1998); Sánchez, *Becoming Mexican American*, pp. 245–49.

107. Natalia Molina, *Fit to Be Citizens? Public Health and Race in Los Angeles, 1879–1940* (Berkeley: University of California Press, 2006).

108. Quoted in Molina, *Fit to Be Citizens?*, p. 172.

109. See Molina, *Fit to Be Citizens?*, pp. 171–75.

110. Quoted in Gutiérrez, *Walls and Mirrors*, p. 113.

111. *Thirty-second Biennial Report of the Department of Public Health*, p. 132.

112. H. Brett Melendy, "Filipinos in the United States," *Pacific Historical Review*, v. 43 (Nov. 1974): 520–47; James D. Sobredo, "From American 'Nationals' to the 'Third Asiatic Invasion': Racial Transformation and Filipino Exclusion (1898–1934)," Ph.D. dissertation, University of California, Berkeley, 1998.

113. See Bruno Lasker, *Filipino Immigration* (Chicago: University of Chicago Press, 1931), pp. 107–15.

114. Benicio Catapusan, "Filipino Immigrants and Public Relief in the United States," *Sociology and Social Research*, v. 23 (July–Aug. 1939): 546–54.

115. Casiano Pagdilao Coloma, "A Study of the Filipino Repatriation Movement," M.A. thesis, School of Social Work, University of Southern California, 1939.

116. Mae M. Ngai, *Impossible Subjects: Illegal Aliens and the Making of Modern America* (Princeton, N.J.: Princeton University Press, 2004).

117. Ronald Takaki, *Strangers from a Different Shore: A History of Asian Americans* (New York: Penguin Books, 1989), p. 333; Sobredo, "From American 'Nationals,'" p. 234.

118. TMR, May 1933.

119. TMR, June 1934. (Presumably the mountain facility housed primarily whites.)

120. TMR, Feb. 1933.

121. Minutes of State Board of Health, April 1933, California State Archives, Sacramento.

122. TMR, May 1933.

123. TMR, May 1933.

124. TMR, Sept. 1933.

125. TMR, Sept. 1933.

126. Cited in Coloma, "Filipino Repatriation Movement," pp. 40–41.

127. A. H. Payne to Board of Supervisors, July 19, 1937, file 40.31/1582, LACBS.

128. Coloma, "Filipino Repatriation Movement," p. 71.

129. Carlos Bulosan, *America Is in the Heart: A Personal History* (Seattle: University of Washington Press, 1943); see Sau-ling Cynthia Wong, *Reading Asian American Literature: From Necessity to Extravagance* (Princeton, N.J.: Princeton University Press, 1993), p. 136.

130. P. C. Morantte, *Remembering Carlos Bulosan* (Los Angeles: Philippine Expressions, 1985), pp. 31–32.

131. See Marilyn Alquizola, "The Fictive Narrator of *America Is in the Heart*," in *Frontiers of Asian American Studies: Writing, Research, and Commentary*, ed. Gail Nomura et al. (Pullman: Washington State University Press, 1989), pp. 211–17; Elaine H. Kim, *Asian American Literature: An Introduction to the Writings and Their Social Context* (Philadelphia: Temple University Press, 1982), pp. 43–57; Rachel C. Lee, *The Americas of Asian American Literature: Gendered Fictions of Nation and Transnation* (Princeton, N.J.: Princeton University Press, 1999), pp. 17–43.

132. Bulosan, *America*, p. 143.

133. Bulosan, *America*, p. 224.

134. Bulosan, *America*, p. 225.

135. Sheila M. Rothman, *Living in the Shadow of Death: Tuberculosis and the Social Experience of Illness in American History* (New York: Basic Books, 1994), p. 228.

136. Bulosan, *America*, p. 225.

137. Bulosan, *America*, p. 54.

138. Bulosan, *America*, p. 226.

139. Bulosan, *America*, p. 147.

140. Bulosan, *America*, p. 147.

141. Bulosan, *America*, p. 232.

142. Robert F. Murphy, *The Body Silent* (New York: W. W. Norton, 1987), p. 57.

143. Bulosan, *America*, p. 251.

144. Bulosan, *America*, p. 247.

145. Bulosan, *America*, p. 238.

146. Bulosan, *America*, p. 255.

147. Bulosan, *America*, p. 240.

148. Bulosan, *America*, p. 252.

149. Bulosan, *America*, p. 246.

150. Bulosan, *America*, p. 232.

151. Bulosan, *America*, p. 236.

152. Bulosan, *America*, p. 236.

153. Bulosan, *America*, p. 246.

154. Bulosan, *America*, pp. 56–57.

155. Bulosan, *America*, p. 237.

156. Bulosan, *America*, pp. 232, 251.

157. Bulosan, *America*, p. 252.

158. Bulosan, *America*, p. 253.

159. Bulosan, *America*, p. 253.

160. Bulosan, *America*, p. 255.

161. See Morantte, *Remembering Carlos Bulosan*, pp. 11–13.

162. Morantte, *Remembering Carlos Bulosan*, p. 11; see also Auguso Fauni Espiritu, "'Expatriate Affirmations': The Performance of Nationalism and Patronage in Filipino-American Intellectual Life," Ph.D. dissertation, University of California, Los Angeles, 2000, pp. 147–49.

Chapter 7 "Agitation over the Migrant Issue"

1. All client names in this chapter are pseudonyms.

2. Council of Social Agencies of Los Angeles, "A Study of Transients Applying for Medical Care at Free and Part-Pay Clinics in Los Angeles," March 10, 1937, no page numbers, file 40.31/1569, LACBS.

3. Council of Social Agencies, "Study of Transients."

4. Council of Social Agencies, "Study of Transients."

5. Council of Social Agencies, "Study of Transients."

6. Council of Social Agencies, "Study of Transients."

7. *Hearings* conducted by the House Select Committee to Investigate the Interstate Migration of Destitute Citizens, Pursuant to H. Res. 63, 491, 629 (76th Congress) and H. Res. 16 (77th Congress) (Washington, D.C., 1941) (hereafter cited as the Tolan Committee), part 6, p. 2236.

8. James N. Gregory, *American Exodus: The Dust Bowl Migration and Okie Culture in California* (New York: Oxford University Press, 1989), p. 83.

9. On attitudes toward both Mexican and African American migrants, see Kenneth L. Kusmer, *Down and Out, on the Road: The Homeless in American History* (New York: Oxford University Press, 2002), p. 223.

10. Gregory, *American Exodus*, p. 42; Walter J. Stein, *California and the Dust Bowl Migration* (Westport, Conn.: Greenwood Press, 1973), pp. 45–46.

11. Tolan Committee, *Hearings*, part 7, p. 2970.

12. John N. Webb and Malcolm Brown, *Migrant Families* (Washington, D.C.: Government Printing Office, 1938), pp. 8, 17.

13. Council of Social Agencies, "Study of Transients."

14. Webb and Brown, *Migrant Families*, p. 8.

15. TMR, July 1934.

16. Interview with David Lubin, Los Angeles, Nov. 3, 2001.

17. Tolan Committee, *Hearings*, part 7, p. 2887.

18. Tolan Committee, *Hearings*, part 6, p. 2458.

19. Council of Social Agencies, "Study of Transients."

20. See *Review of Activities of the State Relief Administration of California, 1933–1935* (San Francisco: State Relief Administration of California, 1936), pp. 93–95; Louis D. Boonshaft, *Medical History and Report, State Relief Administration of California, Los Angeles County* (San Francisco: State Relief Commission, 1937).

21. John L. Pomeroy to Los Angeles County Board of Supervisors, April 8, 1936, file 180/334, LACBS.

22. TMR, July 1938.

23. Zudenka Buben to John L. Pomeroy, Oct. 9, 1933, in Pomeroy, "Administration of Public Health: Viewpoints of Public Health Experts and Los Angeles County Medical Society," p. 86, file 180.3/254, LACBS; Council of Social Agencies, "Study of Transients."

24. Health Department of Los Angeles County, "Annual Reports, Year Ended June 30, 1937," p. 32, file 180.3/414, LACBS.

25. Tolan Committee, *Hearings*, part 6, p. 2237.

26. Tolan Committee, *Hearings*, part 6, p. 2460.

27. *Co-Guilty of Murder? 1939 Annual Report of the Los Angeles Tuberculosis and Health Association* (Los Angeles: Tuberculosis and Health Association, 1938), p. 8.

28. TMR, Sept. 1936.

29. George Parrish, "Letter of Transmittal," in *Annual Report of the Board of Health Commissioners, City of Los Angeles, California, Fiscal Year 1938–39* (Los Angeles: Board of Health Commissioners, 1939), p. 5.

30. TMR, Sept. 1937.

31. See Stein, *Dust Bowl Migration*, p. 119.

32. TMR, Dec. 1938.

33. Edythe Tate-Thompson, "Report of the Bureau of Tuberculosis," in *Thirty-second Biennial Report of the Department of Public Health of California for the Fiscal Years from July 1, 1930, to June 30, 1932* (Sacramento: State Printing Office, 1932), p. 133.

34. TMR, Feb. 1936.

35. John L. Pomeroy to Los Angeles County Board of Supervisors, May 27, 1932, file 180/222, LACBS.

36. TMR, Aug. 1933.

37. TMR, May 1934.

38. Quoted in Richard David Lester, "Building the New Deal State on the Local Level: Unemployment Relief in Los Angeles County during the 1930s," Ph.D. dissertation, University of California, Los Angeles, 2001, p. 288.

39. Gregory, *American Exodus*, p. 80; Kusmer, *Down and Out*, p. 221; Stein, *Dust Bowl Migration*, pp.73–74; Tolan Committee, *Hearings*, part 6, p. 2236.

40. Leonard Joseph Leader, *Los Angeles and the Great Depression*, Ph.D. dissertation, University of California, Los Angeles, 1972, p. 203.

41. TMR, Nov. 1936.

42. Tolan Committee, *Hearings*, part 7, p. 2961.

43. Tolan Committee, *Hearings*, part 7, p. 3035.

44. John L. Pomeroy to Los Angeles County Board of Supervisors, April 8, 1936, file 180/334, LACBS.

45. Health Department of Los Angeles County, "Annual Report, Year Ended June 30, 1936," p. 20, LACBS.

46. TMR, Aug. 1936.

47. TMR, Aug. 1936.

48. TMR, July 1937.

49. Health Department of Los Angeles County, "Annual Report, Year Ended June 30, 1937," p. 2, file 180.3/414, LACBS.

50. Health Department of Los Angeles County, "Annual Report, Year Ended June 30, 1938, p. 97, file 180.3/414.

51. Kusmer, *Down and Out*, pp. 194–95.

52. Tolan Committee, *Hearings*, Part 7, p. 2873; see also Stein, *Dust Bowl Migration*, pp. 116, 126.

53. Tolan Committee, *Hearings*, Part 7, p. 2877.

54. *Summary of Activities of the State Relief Administration Operating in Los Angeles County*, prepared by Saul Pollock (Los Angeles: State Relief Administration, 1940).

55. Rex Thomson to Board of Supervisors, Jan. 23, 1939, file 40.31/1688, LACBS. In 1940, the Department of Charities rejected between 200 and 225 people a month as a result of residency laws. See "Testimony of Lawrence C. Schreiber," Tolan Hearings, part 7, p. 2913.

56. See Los Angeles County Department of Charities, "October Report," 1937, p. 5; "December Report," 1937, p. 8; "February Report," 1938, p. 7; "April Report," 1938, p. 7; "May Report," 1938," p. 6, Box 64, file B 14 c bb aaa, JAF.

57. TMR, Feb. 1936.

58. Letters of A. C. Price and Rex Thomson to Los Angeles County Board of Supervisors, 1933–1938, files 40.31/950–40.31/1645, LACBS.

59. See TMR.

60. Buben to Pomeroy, Oct. 9, 1933.

61. Kusmer, *Down and Out*, pp. 194–95.

62. Case No. A204-731, Council of Social Agencies, "Study of Transients."

63. Case No. A206-899, Council of Social Agencies, "Study of Transients."

64. Case No. 216-570, Council of Social Agencies, "Study of Transients."

65. Case No. A203-867, Council of Social Agencies, "Study of Transients."

66. TMR, April 1934.

67. Gregory, *American Exodus*, p. 48.

68. Edythe Tate-Thompson, "Report of the Bureau of Tuberculosis," in *Thirty-fourth Biennial Report of the Department of Public Health of California for the Fiscal Years from July 1, 1934, to June 30, 1936*, p. 128.

69. Box 12, file 13, Minutes of the Case Committee, JFSS.

70. Box11, file 1, Minutes of Case Committee, JFSS.

71. Box 2, file 2, Minutes of Case Committee, JFSS.

72. TMR, Dec. 1938.

73. TMR, April 1940.

74. Case M53-178E, Council of Social Agencies, "Study of Transients."

75. Minutes of Case Committee, JFSS.

76. See Council of Social Agencies, "Study of Transients"; files 40.31/950–40.31/1645, LACBS.

77. Rex Thomson to Los Angeles County Board of Supervisors, Dec. 10, 1935, file 40.31/1391; Thomson to Board of Supervisors, March 4, 1935, file 40.31/1249; Thomson to Board of Supervisors, June 9, 1936, file 40.31/1434, LACBS.

78. The treatment by state authorities was not unusually harsh. Investigating the condition of migrants returned to California, M. H. Lewis gave the following examples. "A family returned from the state of Washington was sent in a day coach, although a 10-year-old child was so ill that she was unable to sit up; $3 cash to buy food on the journey was allowed in this case. . . . A family returned from Tennessee by bus had an extremely difficult trip. They were delayed by dust storms in Arkansas and Missouri for two days. The man became quite ill. The $5.50 cash which they had been given for food was spent before they had made half the journey." See M. H. Lewis, *Transients in California: Special Surveys and Studies* (San Francisco: State Relief Administration of California, 1936), p. 272.

79. TMR, Dec. 1938.

80. Interview with Frances Feldman, University of Southern California, Los Angeles, Dec. 6, 2002.

81. Rex Thomson to Board of Supervisors, March 25, 1936, file 40.31/1425, LACBS.

82. A. J. Price to Board of Supervisors, Feb. 8, 1934, file 40.31/1028, LACBS.

83. Lewis, *Transients in California*, p. 289.

84. Kusmer, *Down and Out*, p. 223.

85. According to a 1933 report, "the Los Angeles homeless are, for the most part, non-resident men." See *Report and Recommendations of the California State Unemployment Commission* (Sacramento: State Printing Office, 1933), p. 341.

86. Kusmer, *Down and Out*, pp. 206–7.

87. Todd Depastino, *Citizen Hobo: How a Century of Homelessness Shaped America* (Chicago: University of Chicago Press, 2003), p. 209.

88. Council of Social Agencies, "Study of Transients."

89. *State Unemployment Commission*, p. 379.

90. *State Unemployment Commission*, p. 380.

91. Lewis, *Transients in California*, p. 87.

92. TMR, March 1934.

93. TMR, April 1934.

94. TMR, May 1934.

95. See Kusmer, *Down and Out*, pp. 199–201.

96. TMR, July 1934.

97. Lewis, *Transients in California*, p. 97.

98. Lewis, *Transients in California*, p. 97.

99. Rex Thomson to Supervisor John Anson Ford, Dec. 24, 1935, Box 64, file B 14 c bb aaa, JAF.

100. TMR, Jan. 1936.

101. John H. Swan to John Anson Ford, May 28, 1939, Box 64, file B 14 c bb aaa, JAF.

102. E. J. Sneed to George M. Morgan, Feb. 8, 1939, Box 64, file B 14 c bb aaa, JAF.

103. Sneed to Morgan, Feb. 8, 1939.

104. TMR, June 1938.

105. TMR, July 1938.

106. Edythe Tate-Thompson, "Bureau of Tuberculosis, July 1, 1936–June 30, 1938," in *Thirty-fifth Biennial Report of the Department of Public Health of California for the Fiscal Years from July 1, 1936, to June 30, 1938* (Sacramento: State Printing Office, 1938), p. 170.

107. TMR, Feb. 1939.

108. TMR, May 1938.

109. TMR, March 1939.

110. TMR, March 1941.

Chapter 8   Fighting TB in Black Los Angeles

1. See Michael Stewart, "Conclusions: Specters of the Underclass," in *Poverty, Ethnicity, and Gender in Eastern Europe during the Market Transition*, ed. Rebecca Jean Emigh and Iván Szelényi (Westport, Conn.: Praeger, 2001), p. 192.

2. Douglas Flamming, *Bound for Freedom: Black Los Angeles in Jim Crow America* (Berkeley: University of California Press, 2005). As the many footnotes suggest, I draw heavily on this work.

3. Josh Sides, *L.A. City Limits: African American Los Angeles from the Great Depression to the Present* (Berkeley: University of California Press, 2003), p. 15.

4. Quoted in William Deverell and Douglas Flamming, "Race, Rhetoric, and Regional Identity: Boosting Los Angeles, 1880–1930," in *Power and Place in the North American West*, ed. Richard White and John M. Findlay (Seattle: University of Washington Press, 1999), p. 125.

5. Quoted in Deverell and Flamming, "Boosting Los Angeles," p. 126.

6. Quoted in Flamming, *Bound for Freedom*.

7. Flamming, *Bound for Freedom*, p. 51.

8. Flamming, *Bound for Freedom*, p. 76.

9. Sides, *L.A. City Limits*, p. 26.

10. *California Eagle*, Dec. 20, 1919.

11. *California Eagle*, Jan. 7, 1921.

12. *California Eagle*, Aug. 19, 1927.

13. *California Eagle*, April 10, 1931.

14. Darlene Clark Hine, *Black Women in White: Racial Conflict and Cooperation in the Nursing Profession, 1890–1950* (Bloomington: Indiana University Press, 1989), p. 9. The name probably came from the poet Paul Laurence Dunbar.

15. *California Eagle*, Dec. 16, 1927.

16. *California Eagle*, March 6, 1925.

17. National Tuberculosis Association, *A Directory of Sanatoria, Hospitals, Day Camps, and Preventoria for the Treatment of Tuberculosis in the United States* (New York: National Tuberculosis Association, 1923), pp. 9–18.

18. Susan M. Reverby, *Ordered to Care: The Dilemma of American Nursing, 1850–1945* (New York: Cambridge University Press, 1987), p. 61.

19. Hine, *Black Women in White*, p. xv.

20. Hine, *Black Women in White*, p. 6.

21. Helen Eastman Martin, *The History of Los Angeles County Hospital and the Los Angeles County–University of Southern California Medical Center, 1968–1978* (Los Angeles: University of California Press, 1979), p. 28.

22. See Hine, *Black Women in White.*

23. C. H. Whitman to L.A. County Board of Supervisors, Oct. 16, 1911, file OD3436H, LACBS.

24. Petition to Dr. Chas. H. Whitman, Nov. 17, 1911, file OD3447H, LACBS.

25. Petition to the Board of Supervisors, Nov. 18, 1911, file OD3448H, LACBS.

26. L. D. Barnett to L.A. County Board of Supervisors, April 20, 1912, file OD3521H, LACBS.

27. Flamming, *Bound for Freedom*, p. 144.

28. Charlotta A. Bass, *Forty Years: Memoirs from the Pages of a Newspaper* (Los Angeles: Charlotta A. Bass, 1960), p. 47.

29. Quoted in Flamming, *Bound for Freedom*, p. 161.

30. Petition of the Associated Committee to the L.A. County Board of Supervisors, June 24, 1918, file OD4508H, LACBS.

31. Martin, *Los Angeles County Hospital*, p. 47.

32. Quoted in letter of Norman R. Martin to L.A. County Board of Supervisors, July 29, 1918, file OD 4521H, LACBS.

33. Martin to Board of Supervisors, July 29, 1918.

34. *California Eagle*, Sept. 7, 1918.

35. Memo, Jan. 8, 1919, file OD 4603H, LACBS.

36. Letter of E. Burton Ceruti, *California Eagle*, March 22, 1919.

37. *California Eagle*, April 10, 1931.

38. *California Eagle*, Feb. 3, 1928.

39. See *California Eagle*, Nov. 31, 1938; Floyd C. Covington, "Political Activity Schedule," May 25, 1940, Box 2, file 16, LAUL; Covington to T. Arnold Hill, Feb. 3, 1940, Box 2, file 16, LAUL.

40. *California Eagle*, Oct. 13, 1933.

41. *California Eagle*, Oct. 13, 1933.

42. Helen Bruce, "Occupations for Negro Women in Los Angeles," May 28, 1933, pp. 7–8, Box 1, file F.2, LAUL.

43. *California Eagle*, April 13, 1934.

44. *California Eagle*, July 20, 1939.

45. *California Eagle*, Feb. 23, 1956.

46. Flamming, *Bound for Freedom*, p. 40.

47. Quoted in Tera W. Hunter, *To "Joy My Freedom": Southern Black Women's Lives and Labors after the Civil War* (Cambridge, Mass.: Harvard University Press, 1997), p. 196.

48. Nancy Tomes, *The Gospel of Germs: Men, Women, and the Microbe in American Life* (Cambridge, Mass.: Harvard University Press, 1998), pp. 222–33.

49. *California Eagle*, Feb. 23, 1956.

50. TMR, July 1934.

51. TMR, Nov. 1934. Some of their opposition appears to have stemmed from anger at the interference of state officials.

52. TMR, Aug. 1935.

53. TMR, March 1939.

54. See Tomes, *Gospel of Germs*, p. 231.

55. "Report of the Executive Secretary for March 1933," GPC.

56. "Report of the Executive Secretary for June 1933," GPC.

57. Quoted in Beatrix Hoffman, *The Wages of Sickness: The Politics of Health Insurance in Progressive America* (Chapel Hill: University of North Carolina Press, 2001), p. 61. See Samuel Robers, "Infectious Fear: Tuberculosis, Public Health, and the Logic of Race and Illness in Baltimore, Maryland, 1880–1930," Ph.D. dissertation, Princeton University, Nov. 2002.

58. Hoffman, *Wages of Sickness*, pp. 60–61; Katherine Ott, *Fevered Lies: Tuberculosis in American Culture since 1870* (Cambridge, Mass.: Harvard University Press, 1996), 100–110; Marion Torchia, "Tuberculosis among American Negroes: Medical Research on a Racial Disease," *Journal of the History of Medicine*, v. 32 (1977): 252–79.

59. *California Eagle*, April 3, 1931.

60. "Report of the Executive Secretary for February 1935," GPC.

61. Susan L. Smith, *Sick and Tired of Being Sick and Tired: Black Women's Health Activism in America, 1890–1950* (Philadelphia: University of Pennsylvania Press, 1995), p. 58.

62. *California Eagle*, March 31, 1933.

63. "Report of the Board of Directors, Los Angeles Tuberculosis and Health Association," Jan. 22, 1939, Breathe California of Los Angeles County, Los Angeles.

64. Flamming, *Bound for Freedom*, pp. 242–47.

65. See Hine, *Black Women in White*, p. 59.

66. "Report of Board of Directors," Aug. 23, 1938.

67. *1938: Annual Report of the Los Angeles Tuberculosis and Health Association*, p. 5.

68. "Report of Board of Directors," Nov. 27, 1938.

69. "Report of Board of Directors," Aug. 23, 1938.

70. *California Eagle*, July 18, 1940.

71. *California Eagle*, May 6, 1916.

72. Flamming, *Bound for Freedom*, p. 25.

73. *California Eagle*, May 6, 1916.

74. *California Eagle*, Oct. 14, 1922.

75. *California Eagle*, Aug. 17, 1923.

76. Flamming, *Bound for Freedom*, pp. 226–42, 296–364.

77. *California Eagle*, Aug. 22, 1934; Sides, *L.A. City Limits*, p. 27.

78. *California Eagle*, 1934–1940.

79. Quoted in Flamming, *Bound for Freedom*, p. 104.

80. *California Eagle*, Feb. 1, 1940.

81. Bass, *Forty Years*, p. 27.

82. *California Eagle*, Jan. 5, 1939.

83. *California Eagle*, July 21, 1938.

84. TMR, Dec. 1940.

85. *California Eagle*, July 11, 1940.

86. *California Eagle*, June 20, 1940, July 18, 1940.

Epilogue

1. Léopold Banc and Mukund Uplekar, "The Present Global Burden of Tuberculosis," in *The Return of the White Plague: Global Poverty and the "New" Tuberculosis*, ed. Matthew Gandy and Alimuddin Zumla (New York: Verso, 2003), p. 95; Henry M. Blumberg, Michael K. Leonard, and Robert M. Jasmer, "Update on the Treatment of Tuberculosis and Latent Tuberculosis Infection," *Journal of the American Medical Association (JAMA)*, v. 293, no. 22 (June 8, 2005): 2776.

2. Mary D. Nettleman, "Multidrug-Resistant Tuberculosis: News from the Front," *JAMA*, v. 293, no. 22 (June 8, 2005): 2726–32.

3. Banc and Uplekar, "Global Burden," p. 95.

4. Quoted in "International AIDS Conference 2006: Treat TB to Keep People with AIDS Alive" (Aug. 9, 2006), http://www.results.org/website/article.asp?id=2330.

5. Banc and Uplekar, "Global Burden," p. 95; Maria Cheng, "Experts Urge Fight against TB in Africa" (Sept. 12, 2006), http://www.wtop.com/?nid=106&sid=909856.

6. Donald G. McNeil, Jr., "TB Declines, but Not in Immigrants," *New York Times*, March 22, 2005, p. D2; Donald G. McNeil, Jr., "Tuberculosis Declines to Historic Low in the U.S.," *New York Times*, March 24, 2006, p. A11.

7. "Bitter Harvest: Migrant Worker Health," *UC Mexus News*, no. 42 (Summer 2005): 6–9.

8. McNeil, "TB Declines," p. D2.

9. Madeleine Pelner Cosman, "Illegal Aliens and American Medicine," *Journal of American Physicians and Surgeons*, v. 10, no. 1 (Spring 2005): 6.

10. David D. Kirkpatrick, "Demonstrations on Immigration Harden a Divide," *New York Times*, April 17, 2006, p. A1.

11. Solomon Moore, "L.A. Fights to Cure TB One Case at a Time," *Los Angeles Times*, July 11, 2005, p. A1.

12. See Nina Bernstein, "Recourse Grows Slim for Immigrants Who Fall Ill," *New York Times*, March 3, 2006, p. Al.

13. Bernstein, "Recourse Grows Slim."

14. "Illegal Aliens Putting Strain on Hospitals," Lou Dobbs Show, CNN, April 8, 2005 (transcript).

15. Dana Canedy, "Hospitals Feeling Strain from Illegal Immigrants," *New York Times*, Aug. 25, 2002, p. A12.

16. Mrs. K. G. to F.D.R., Missouri, May 11, 1939, file 4-9-1-1, Children's Bureau Records, National Archives, Washington, D.C.

Index

About the Author

Emily K. Abel is professor of health services and women's studies at University of California, Los Angeles. Her most recent books are *Hearts of Wisdom: American Women Caring for Kin, 1850–1940* (Harvard University Press, 2000), and *Suffering in the Land of Sunshine: A Los Angeles Illness Narrative* (Rutgers University Press, 2006).